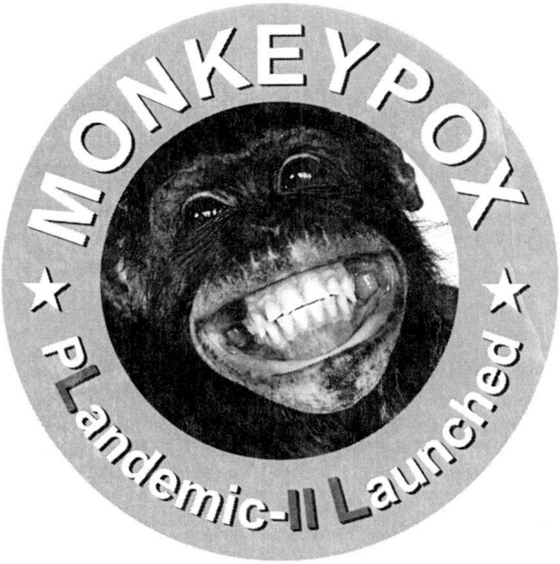

DR. BISWAROOP ROY CHOWDHURY

DIAMOND BOOKS

India Office:
C/o India Book of Records
B-121, 2nd Floor, Greenfields,
Faridabad -120003 (Haryana),
India
Ph.: +91-9312286540

Malaysia Office:
C/o Bishwaroop International Healing & Research
PT 573, Lot 15077 Jalan Tuanku
Munawir,
70000 Negeri Sembilan, Malaysia
Tel: +6012-2116089

Vietnam Office:
C/o Vietnam Book of Records
148 Hong Ha Street
9 Award, Phu Nhuan District,
Ho Chi Minh City, Vietnam
- Hotline: (+84) 903710505

Switzerland Office:
C/o Nigel Kingsley
Kraftwerkstr. 95, ch-5465, Mellikon,
Switzerland
Tel: 0041 79 222 2323

FOLLOW ME

Facebook: https://www.facebook.com/drbrc.official/
Twitter: https://twitter.com/drbrcofficial
Bitchute: https://www.bitchute.com/channel/drbiswarooproychowdhury/
Instagram: https://www.instagram.com/dr.biswarooproychowdhury/
Telegram: https://t.me/drbiswarooproychowdhury
Email: biswaroop@biswaroop.com
Website: www.biswaroop.com
Video Channel: www.coronakaal.tv

Research : Rachna Sharma
Graphics Designer: Shankar Singh Koranga
Copy Editor: Sanjana Bhowmick

Published by
Diamond Pocket Books
X-30, Okhla Industrial Area, New Delhi-110020
Ph: 011-40712100 email: sales@dpb.in website: www.diamondbook.in

Dedication

Dedicated to my angel daughter Ivy,

loving wife Neerja

&

caring parents

Shri Bikash Roy Chowdhury

Shrimati Lila Roy Chowdhury

Contents

Unveiling Monkeypox Virus

How can we save ourselves from Monkeypox? Or we should say how can we save ourselves from the game of Monkeypox. As a matter of fact using the name of a monkey, as an excuse you are being made a fool or as the idiom goes, a donkey. At the outset, why should you believe in what I have to say ?

Let me explain. Try and recall the time of the year in January 2020. We all watched the coverage on the so called Wuhan's mysterious virus on television like a spine-chilling scary movie. The same was being written by all the leading newspapers of our country as it was across the world.

This was the time when through various national and international media platforms like The Statesman, Dainik Bhaskar, Gulf News, YouTube and other social media, I tried to warn and explain that a game is about to begin in our nation. A simple cold, cough, and fever will be given the shape and form of a pandemic, and it will end only after the human population takes repeated doses of vaccines. And this is exactly what you witnessed during the course of time.

At the same time, I tried to elucidate to you the fact that this is a regular flu and that anyway every year we see the occurrence of influenza. The treatment for the same is a simple three-step flu diet which includes an intake of coconut water and citrus fruit juices. Within a span of three days anyone can easily be cured out of this seasonal flu.

In the beginning of 2020 Dr. Biswaroop alerted the world through national/international media.

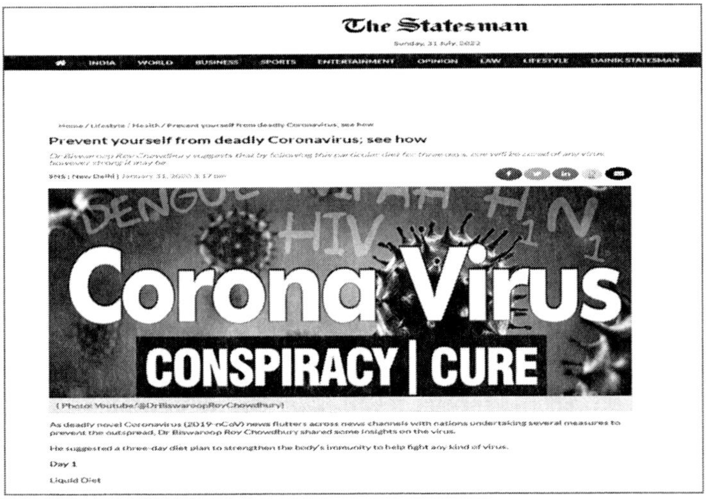

The Statesman

Sunday, 31 July, 2022

INDIA WORLD BUSINESS SPORTS ENTERTAINMENT OPINION LAW LIFESTYLE DAINIK STATESMAN

Home / Lifestyle / Health / Prevent yourself from deadly Coronavirus; see how

Prevent yourself from deadly Coronavirus; see how

SNS | New Delhi | January 31, 2020 3:17 pm

(Photo: Youtube/@DrBiswaroopRoyChowdhury)

As deadly novel Coronavirus (2019-nCoV) news flutters across news channels with nations undertaking several measures to prevent the outspread, Dr Biswaroop Roy Chowdhury shared some insights on the virus.

He suggested a three-day diet plan to strengthen the body's immunity to help fight any kind of virus.

Day 1

Liquid Diet

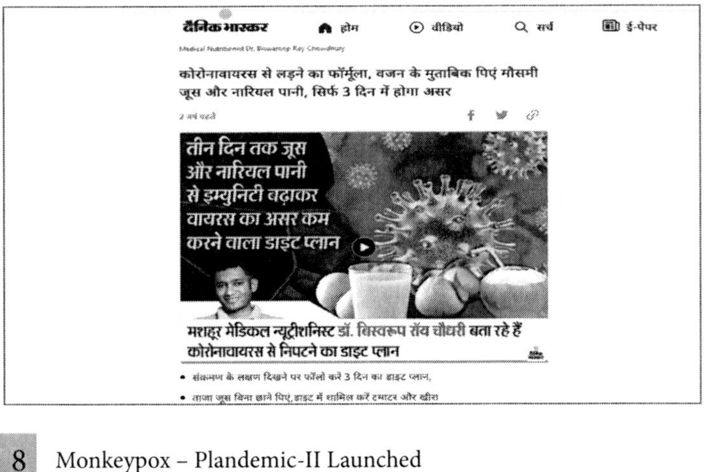

दैनिक भास्कर होम वीडियो सर्च ई-पेपर

कोरोनावायरस से लड़ने का फॉर्मूला, वजन के मुताबिक पिएं मौसमी जूस और नारियल पानी, सिर्फ 3 दिन में होगा असर

मशहूर मेडिकल न्यूट्रीशनिस्ट डॉ. बिस्वरूप रॉय चौधरी बता रहे हैं कोरोनावायरस से निपटने का डाइट प्लान

- संक्रमण के लक्षण दिखने पर फॉलो करें 3 दिन का डाइट प्लान,
- ताजा जूस बिना छाने पिएं, डाइट में शामिल करें टमाटर और खीरा

MENU | World | UAE | Opinion | Dhuhr 12:28

World
ASIA

Gulf News

India | Pakistan | Philippines

COVID-19: Vitamin C, herd immunity the hope for India, Indian doctor says

Delhi-based nutritionist says WHO protocol for treatment of virus is extremely harsh

Published: April 03, 2020
Gautam Bhattacharyya, Senior Associate Editor

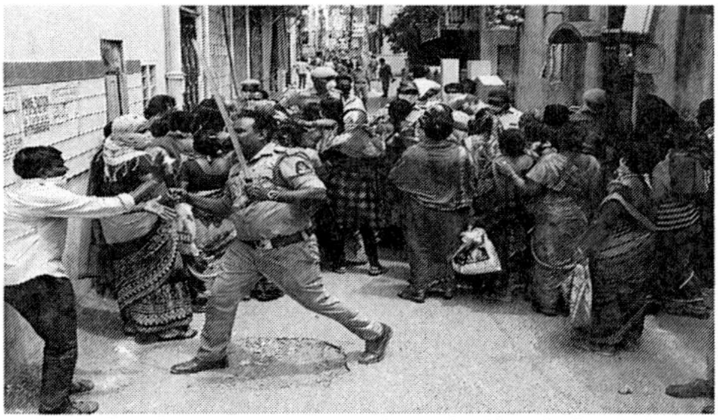

A policeman tries to disburse people who gathered without maintaining social distancing in Hyderabad during the nationwide lockdown earlier week. The herd immunity among the huge population, doctors hope, can slow down the coronavirus pandemic.
Image Credit: ANI

Dubai: A New Delhi-based Indian doctor says that a simple 'preventive diet' to boost the immunity against flu, along with the possibility of the herd immunity already kicking in - may work for the second-most populous country in the world in their fight against the coronavirus pandemic.

Dr Biswaroop Roy Chowdhury - a medical nutritionist whose crash diet plans to reverse diabetes recently became hugely popular via youtube videos - has provided some food for thought at a time when the COVID-19 pandemic has brought the world to it's knees.

Speaking to Gulf News during an exclusive interview, Dr Roy Chowdhury said that in the absence of a vaccine, it's the " treatment and not the disease" which is taking more lives around the world. "Check the WHO protocol and you will see it's a combination of anti-malarial, antibiotics, anti-pyretic and even in cases a HIV drug. Why do you need antibiotics to treat what is essentially a viral fever? Even the dosage of anti-pyretic is also extremely high and it can often turn out to be a lethal combination," he said.

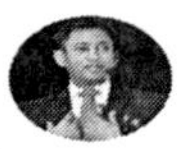

> **Check the WHO protocol and you will see it's a combination of anti-malarial, antibiotics, anti-pyretic and even in cases a HIV drug. Why do you need antibiotics to treat what is essentially a viral fever? Even the dosage of anti-pyretic is also extremely high and it can often turn out to be a lethal combination"**
>
> - Dr Biswaroop Roy Chowdhury

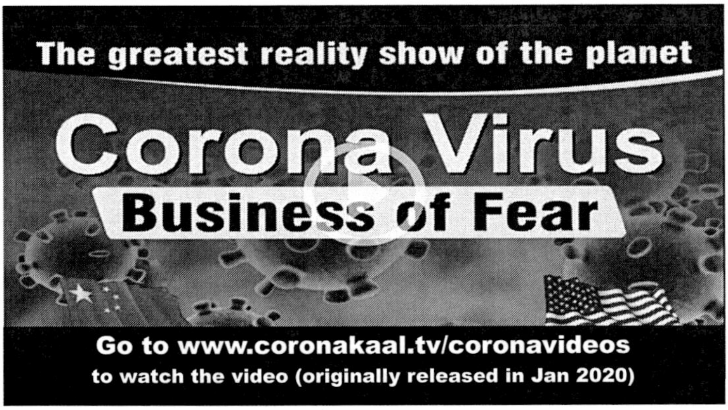

In fact, in the next three to four months, I proved with evidence by curing the first 5000 COVID-19 patients who were nothing but patients with influenza. Thereafter, I released the book, 'N.I.C.E Way to Cure Covid-19' which was a best seller on Amazon for a prolonged period. Though it was strange that this book mysteriously vanished from the Amazon Book Store.

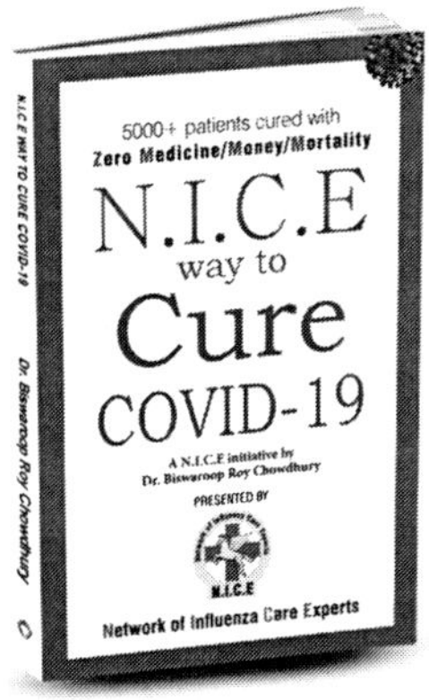

Next, we opened COVID-19 centres (we call it a flu centre) at various locations. Of these, the Ahmednagar Covid-19 Centre became very popular where we successfully proved that even the most difficult of Covid-19 patients, that actually were the flu patients, easily recovered with coconut water and citrus fruit juice.

Glimpses of Ahmednagar Covid-19 Centre

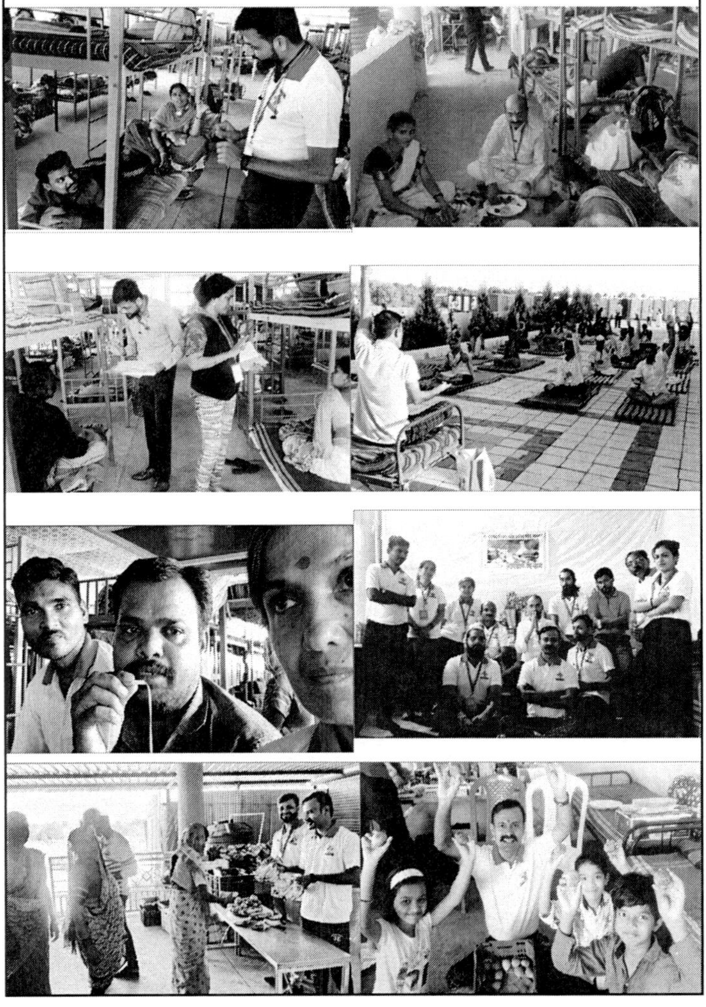

As you can see in the picture, despite treating thousands of patients, we reported no social distancing, no sanitizer, no mask, no PPE Kit, no oxygen cylinder, no medication, no side-effect, and no death.

So much so that the National Institute of Naturopathy (NIN), Ministry of AYUSH conducted a three month observational study on our treatment methodology. After three months they rolled out their report wherein they mentioned and agreed to the fact, that with our three-step flu-diet, even the most difficult or critical of the Covid-19 patients, whom we call as flu patients, can be successfully treated and recovered.

राष्ट्रीय प्राकृतिक चिकित्सा संस्थान, पुणे
आयुष मंत्रालय, भारत सरकार
NATIONAL INSTITUTE OF NATUROPATHY
Ministry of AYUSH, Govt. of India
'Bapu Bhavan' Matoshree Ramabai Ambedkar Road, Pune 411 001
Email:ninpune@bharatmail.co.in | Website: www.ninpune.ayush.gov.in
Phone: 020-26059682 / 3 / 4 / 5 Fax: 020-26059131

NIN-Report on Observational Study on 3 Step Flu Diet

NIN mentioned that in future for similar cases, our three step flu diet can be recommended to patients. This includes dosage of coconut water and citrus fruit juices, which we refer to as the N.I.C.E Protocol.

Highlights of NIN, Ministry of Ayush Study:

1. With N.I.C.E Protocol (flu diet) most of the patients got cured in 7 days
2. No medicine was given
3. No side effects were observed
4. No death occurred
5. Even severe patients were cured successfully

In this way we could successfully prove that what is being highlighted and propagated as Covid-19, is in reality nothing but regular influenza or flu. It is not a contagious disease and there is no need to follow any of the conventional protocols advised by the WHO like wearing of masks, social distancing, using PPE Kits etc.

The question that repeatedly arises in the minds of people is that, if this was not a pandemic, but merely a game, then how did we see lakhs of Covid-19 deaths across the world?

In order to answer this question, we conducted an experiment. We collected various non-human samples like insects, birds, animals like rabbits, rats, dogs, fruits, and even vegetables.

Non-human sample for RT-PCR testing for Covid-19

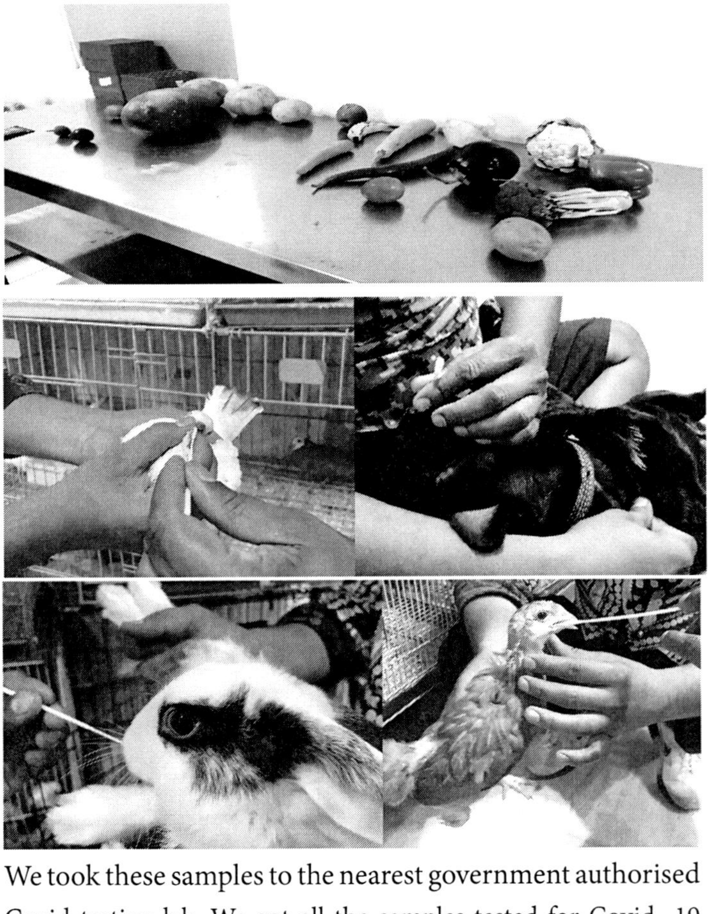

We took these samples to the nearest government authorised Covid-testing lab. We got all the samples tested for Covid -19 in the RT-PCR machine and shockingly, the results for all the samples were positive. As per our calculation, we

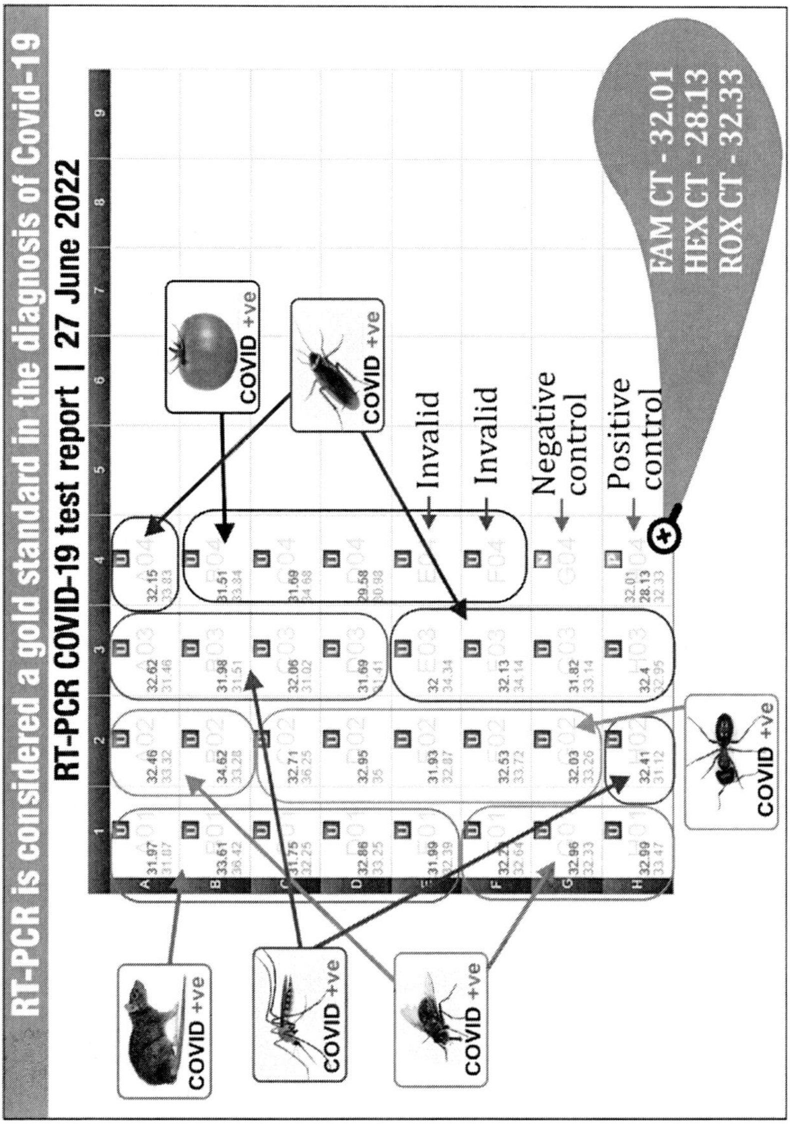
RT-PCR is considered a gold standard in the diagnosis of Covid-19
RT-PCR COVID-19 test report | 27 June 2022
COVID +ve
COVID +ve
COVID +ve
COVID +ve
COVID +ve
COVID +ve
Invalid
Invalid
Negative control
Positive control
FAM CT - 32.01
HEX CT - 28.13
ROX CT - 32.33

concluded that if we take any sample and run through the RT-PCR Covid-19 test machine, then in every 10 tests of the same sample, one result is most likely to be tested as positive. So at any given time if we want to give a nationwide figure that currently we have one lakh Covid-19 cases across the country, then all we need to do is to conduct 10 lakh Covid-19 tests. It is not necessary that these tests need to be conducted using samples of people who are ill and suffering with Covid-19 or flu-like symptoms. We can use the samples of a healthy individual as well. Moreover, even that is not a mandate, as we can take samples of almost any species of fruits, vegetables, birds or animals that we can find around us.

To know the details about the tests and test reports, read the book 'Naked Truth of Covid Test' available at this link on my website: www.biswaroop.com/ebooks

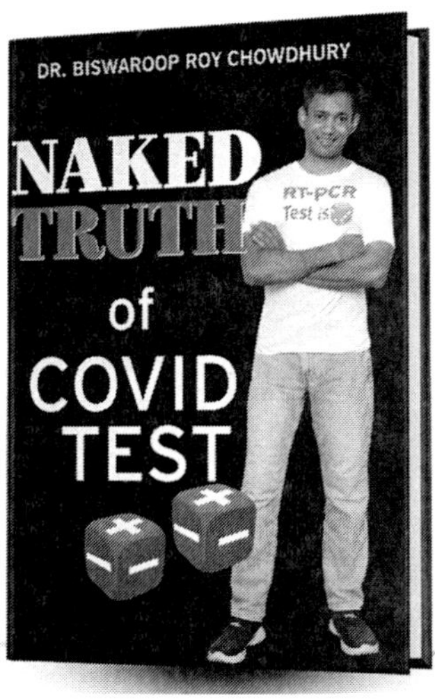

It is easy to understand that we can take any human and convince him that he is Covid-19 positive at any given time. From the same population the ones who

are scared or unwell (because of comorbid conditions) or those who rush to a hospital for treatment, they are then administered with dangerous and poisonous medicines like Remdesivir, Lopinavir, Ritonavir & Plasma Therapy. With high doses of these lethal drugs/treatment protocols some people succumb and are then declared as patients who died of Covid-19.

As a result, when medicines like Remdesivir, which were popularised as the elixir, started adversely affecting the health of individuals and people started dying due to its intake. Hence, Remdesivir was quietly taken off the market and declared as a banned drug.

So as part of this game, basic maladies like cold, cough, and fever were sensationalised and given the proportion of a pandemic.

The planning for the same had been done well in advances which can be proved by the fact that in October 2019 the Bill and Melinda Gates Foundation conducted a drill titled **'Event 201'**. In case you want to go through the detailed video and other documentation, then you can visit the link-

www.biswaroop.com/pandemichoax

The modus operandi remains the same, however this time, instead of cold, cough, and fever, the symptoms chosen were boils, pimples, and heat rashes. Efforts are now being made

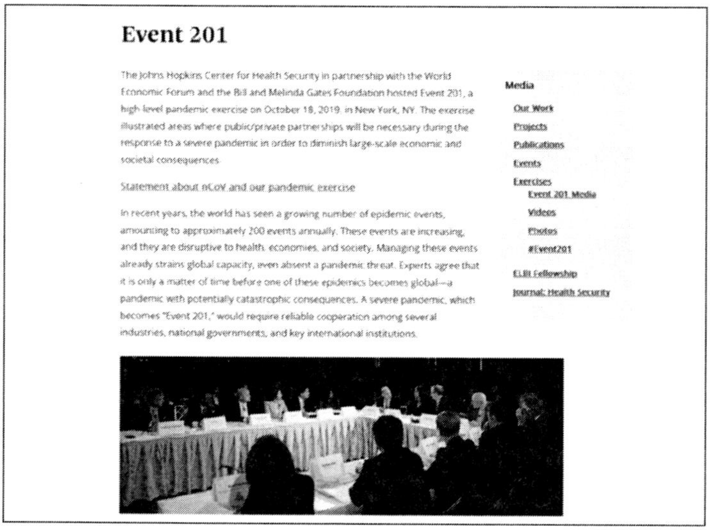
Event 201

The Johns Hopkins Center for Health Security in partnership with the World Economic Forum and the Bill and Melinda Gates Foundation hosted Event 201, a high-level pandemic exercise on October 18, 2019, in New York, NY. The exercise illustrated areas where public/private partnerships will be necessary during the response to a severe pandemic in order to diminish large-scale economic and societal consequences.

Statement about nCoV and our pandemic exercise

In recent years, the world has seen a growing number of epidemic events, amounting to approximately 200 events annually. These events are increasing, and they are disruptive to health, economies, and society. Managing these events already strains global capacity, even absent a pandemic threat. Experts agree that it is only a matter of time before one of these epidemics becomes global—a pandemic with potentially catastrophic consequences. A severe pandemic, which becomes "Event 201," would require reliable cooperation among several industries, national governments, and key international institutions.

Media

Our Work

Projects

Publications

Events

Exercises

Event 201 Media

Videos

Photos

#Event201

ELBI Fellowship

Journal: Health Security

to declare these as a large scale pandemic called Monkeypox. The planning for the next pandemic was has already been executed as early as March 2021.

In March 2021, **'Nuclear Threat Initiative' (NTI)** which is a WHO sponsored organisation, conducted a mock drill to identify how the next pandemic takes a shape or how they can play the next game called Monkeypox. Thereafter, in November 2021, they secretly released documentation. I have been able to get my hands on a copy of that secret documentation as shown next. You can get this document through the link: www.biswaroop.com/pandemichoax

This copy contains the step-by-step details regarding staging a fake Monkeypox pandemic. It contains details of how and till when the game of pandemic would last. In addition, the document states in detail how many people will die of Monkeypox, and how they will succumb to this so-called disease.

Let us dig deep into this document.

Here you can see the first page of the document.

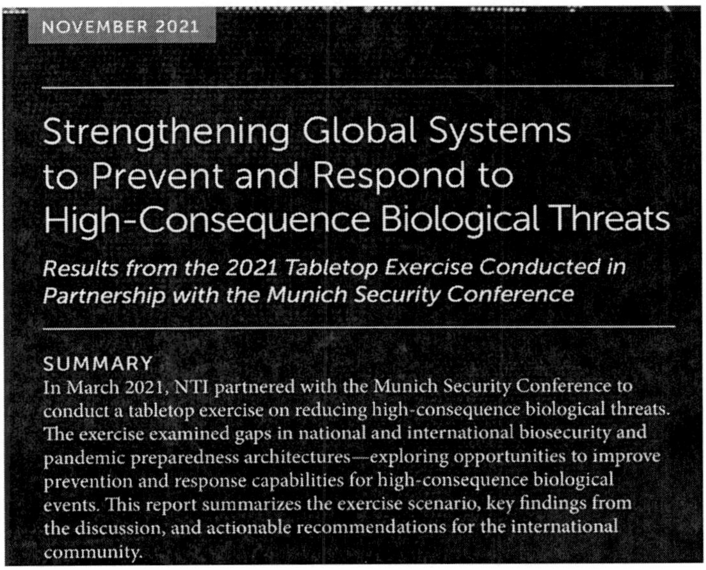

NOVEMBER 2021

Strengthening Global Systems to Prevent and Respond to High-Consequence Biological Threats

Results from the 2021 Tabletop Exercise Conducted in Partnership with the Munich Security Conference

SUMMARY

In March 2021, NTI partnered with the Munich Security Conference to conduct a tabletop exercise on reducing high-consequence biological threats. The exercise examined gaps in national and international biosecurity and pandemic preparedness architectures—exploring opportunities to improve prevention and response capabilities for high-consequence biological events. This report summarizes the exercise scenario, key findings from the discussion, and actionable recommendations for the international community.

Page 1 of document released by NTI

Moving ahead we see the planning on how the media will cover the news.

Check the image given below and pay attention to the date it mentions i.e May 10, 2023. This means that starting from July, 2022 through to the next year 2023, how will the news channels spread the details about Monkeypox, the preparation towards the same in the form of the mock drill has already been accomplished.

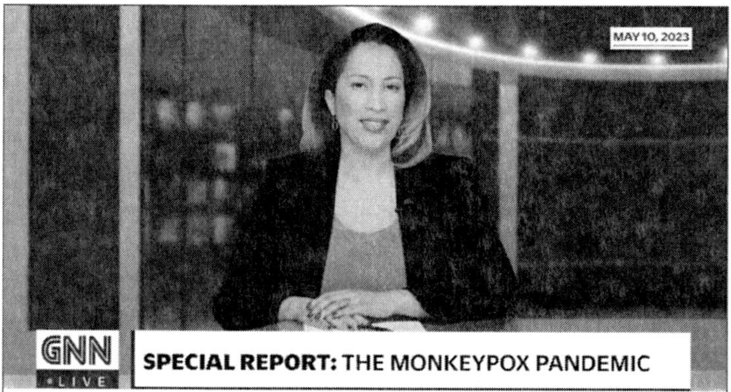

The fictional exercise scenario unfolded in a series of short news videos that participants reacted to.

Let me share a small pattern pertaining to the same. Here is a sample of the news and information shared about Monkeypox currently across the newspapers.

The following pic is a clipping from the newspaper, the **'Times of India'** dated May 22, 2022, that was released across the nation.

Printed from
THE TIMES OF INDIA

Doctors now urge to be alert about Monkeypox

TNN | May 22, 2022, 04.41 AM IST

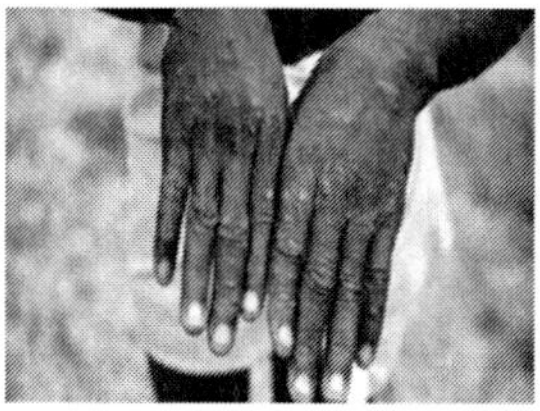

NEW DELHI: The Covid-19 pandemic isn't over yet. But there already are reports of another viral infection called monkeypox spreading in Europe. No such case has been reported in India yet.
The first case of the viral infection in humans, which otherwise infects simians, was reported in 1970 in the Democratic Republic of the Congo. Infectious disease experts say there have been very few cases of monkeypox outside central and west Africa in the past 50 years. That's why the sudden spread of the disease in Europe in unusually high numbers has raised an alarm. The World Health Organization has called an emergency meeting to discuss the outbreak.

ALSO READ
Explainer: What is monkeypox, symptoms and how it spreads

Congratulations!

You have successfully cast your vote

Login to view result

In India, the Union health ministry has directed the National Centre for Disease Control and Indian Council of Medical Research to keep a close watch on the outbreak. Also, if cases continue to increase, the government could start random screening of people arriving from the affected nations.

Here, in the news article it was made to believe that people have already started getting affected by Monkeypox which results in boils and pimples on their body as seen in the image. The article elucidates details about the same. In reality there is no truth to it. The image has been taken from the **'old archives'** for the purpose of this article. Similar instances have been observed quite a number of times over the past few months where the same image has been used.

For instance, the same image appeared in the **'The Sun'** dated September 11, 2018 in another context.

THE Sun

Sign in

UK Edition   Search

MONEY HEALTH DEAR DEIDRE TECH TRAVEL MOTORS PUZZLES SUN BINGO SUN VOUCHERS VISUAL STORIES TOPICS

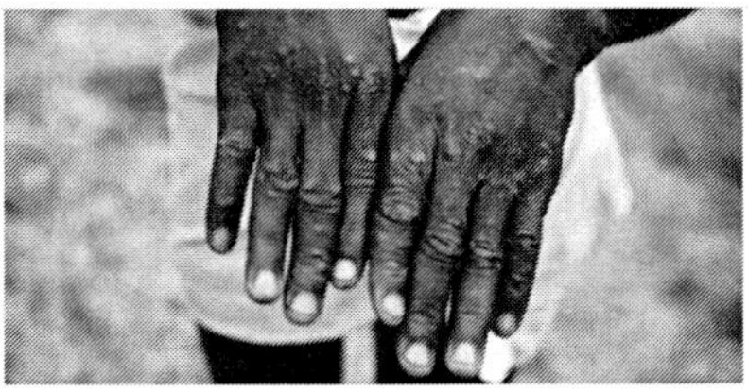

News > Health News

KILLER VIRUS Monkeypox outbreak fears grow as second case of deadly disease confirmed in UK

Monkeypox can cause fever, headache, muscle aches, backache, swollen lymph nodes, chills and exhaustion

Andrea Downey

17:13, 11 Sep 2018   Updated: 19:38, 11 Sep 2018

A SECOND case of monkeypox has been recorded in the UK, health bosses warned today.

It is believed the patient contracted the infection while travelling in Nigeria.

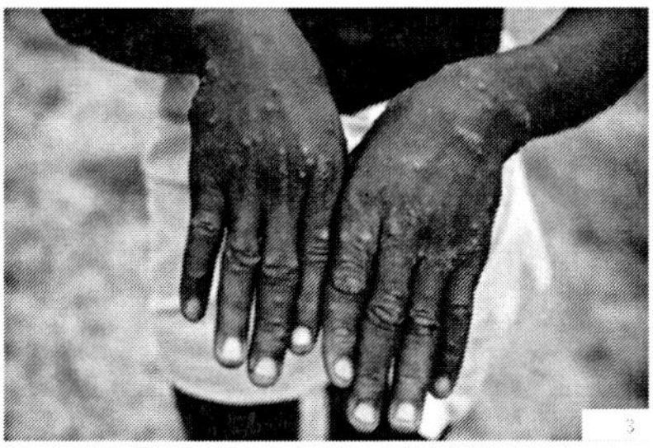

A second case of monkeypox has been confirmed in the UK Credit: Alamy

They first presented at Blackpool Victoria Hospital and, following a positive test result, was transferred to Royal Liverpool University Hospital, an expert respiratory infectious disease centre, where they are receiving appropriate care, Public Health England (PHE) said today.

Over the weekend more than 50 people were warned they may have been

Similarly, the **'BBC'** published this image on December 21, 2017

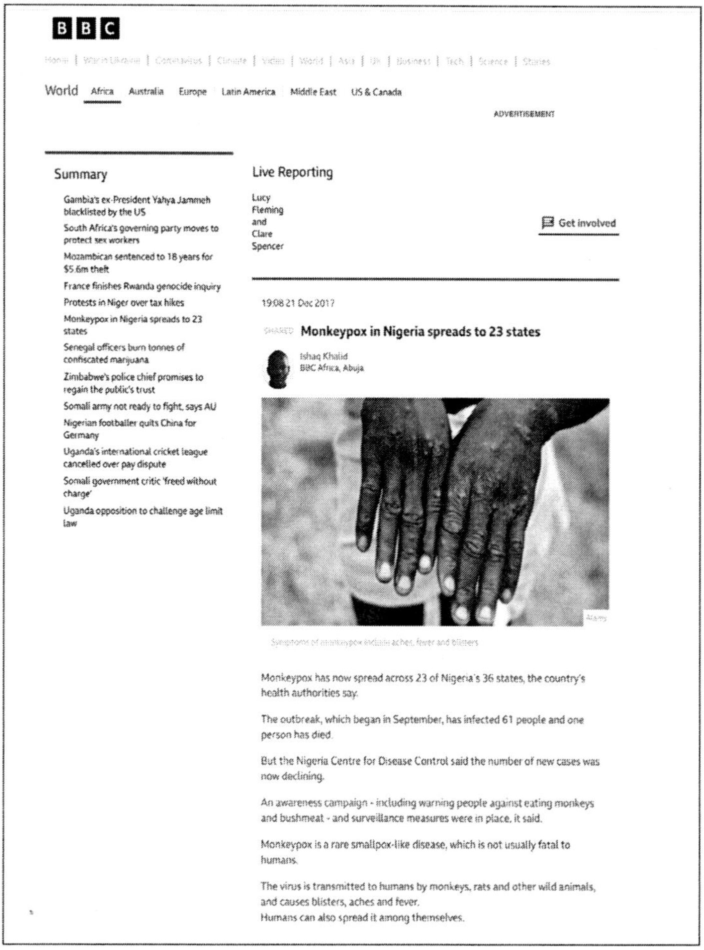

BBC

Home | War in Ukraine | Coronavirus | Climate | Video | World | Asia | UK | Business | Tech | Science | Stories

World Africa Australia Europe Latin America Middle East US & Canada

ADVERTISEMENT

Summary

- Gambia's ex-President Yahya Jammeh blacklisted by the US
- South Africa's governing party moves to protect sex workers
- Mozambican sentenced to 18 years for $5.6m theft
- France finishes Rwanda genocide inquiry
- Protests in Niger over tax hikes
- Monkeypox in Nigeria spreads to 23 states
- Senegal officers burn tonnes of confiscated marijuana
- Zimbabwe's police chief promises to regain the public's trust
- Somali army not ready to fight, says AU
- Nigerian footballer quits China for Germany
- Uganda's international cricket league cancelled over pay dispute
- Somali government critic 'freed without charge'
- Uganda opposition to challenge age limit law

Live Reporting

Lucy Fleming and Clare Spencer

Get involved

19:08 21 Dec 2017

SHARED **Monkeypox in Nigeria spreads to 23 states**

Ishaq Khalid
BBC Africa, Abuja

Alamy

Symptoms of monkeypox include aches, fever and blisters

Monkeypox has now spread across 23 of Nigeria's 36 states, the country's health authorities say.

The outbreak, which began in September, has infected 61 people and one person has died.

But the Nigeria Centre for Disease Control said the number of new cases was now declining.

An awareness campaign - including warning people against eating monkeys and bushmeat - and surveillance measures were in place, it said.

Monkeypox is a rare smallpox-like disease, which is not usually fatal to humans.

The virus is transmitted to humans by monkeys, rats and other wild animals, and causes blisters, aches and fever.
Humans can also spread it among themselves.

And if you want to further find references to this image, it can be found in the Archives dated January 1, 1997.

Search the world's best editorial photos

Monkeypox Lesions

Close-up of monkeypox lesions on the hands of a patient during the recuperative stage of the virus. Democratic Republic of the Congo, 1997. Courtesy CDC/Mahy et al. (Photo via Smith Collection/Gado/Getty Images)

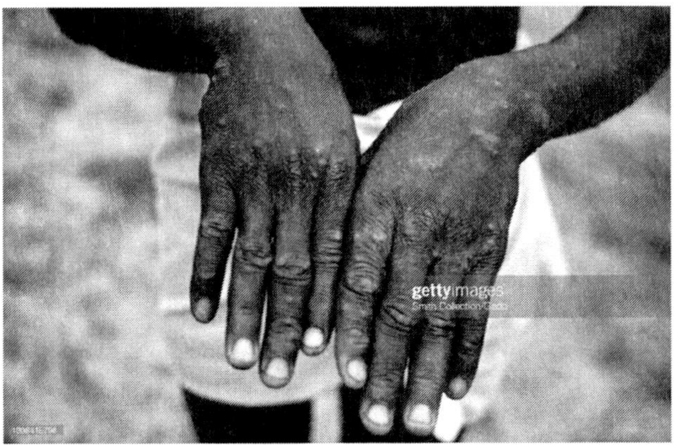

Please note: images depicting historical events may contain themes, or have descriptions, that do not reflect current understanding. They are provided in a historical context. Learn more.

DETAILS

Restrictions:	Contact your local office for all commercial or promotional uses.
Credit:	Smith Collection/Gado / Contributor
Editorial #:	1398415798
Collection:	Archive Photos
Date created:	01 January, 1997
Licence type:	Rights-managed
Release info:	Not released. More information
Source:	Archive Photos
Object name:	285436final
Max file size:	5400 x 3547 px (45.72 x 30.03 cm) - 300 dpi - 8 MB

More fr

Evidently, the efforts are being made towards scaring the general public by the display of an old photograph from the archives.

Moving ahead, let us take a look at the next image that is being used rampantly by the media of late. You must have easily identified this image where it seems that this is the reality of how Monkeypox symptoms appear on the bodies of patients. The reality, however, is far from the truth. The image being used is not current and not of a Monkeypox patient. It is an old archived image of November 2010.

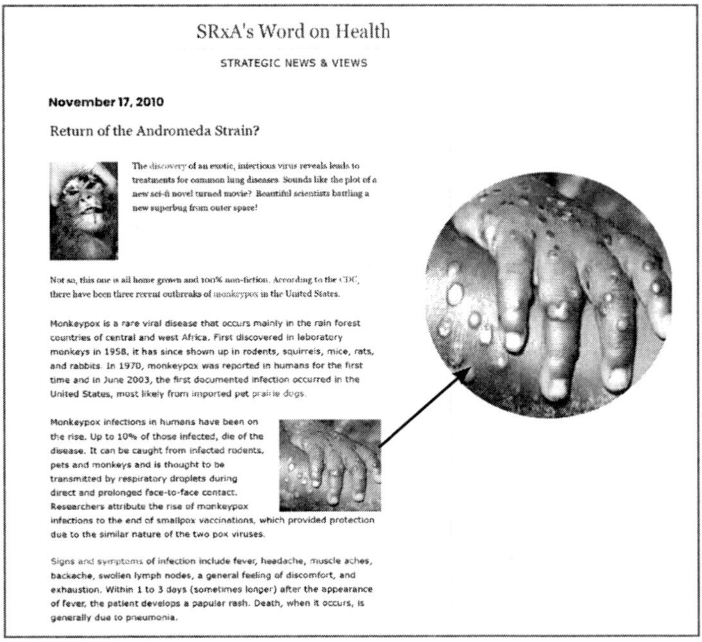

SRxA's Word on Health

STRATEGIC NEWS & VIEWS

November 17, 2010

Return of the Andromeda Strain?

The discovery of an exotic, infectious virus reveals leads to treatments for common lung diseases. Sounds like the plot of a new sci-fi novel turned movie? Beautiful scientists battling a new superbug from outer space!

Not so, this one is all home grown and 100% non-fiction. According to the CDC, there have been three recent outbreaks of monkeypox in the United States.

Monkeypox is a rare viral disease that occurs mainly in the rain forest countries of central and west Africa. First discovered in laboratory monkeys in 1958, it has since shown up in rodents, squirrels, mice, rats, and rabbits. In 1970, monkeypox was reported in humans for the first time and in June 2003, the first documented infection occurred in the United States, most likely from imported pet prairie dogs.

Monkeypox infections in humans have been on the rise. Up to 10% of those infected, die of the disease. It can be caught from infected rodents, pets and monkeys and is thought to be transmitted by respiratory droplets during direct and prolonged face-to-face contact. Researchers attribute the rise of monkeypox infections to the end of smallpox vaccinations, which provided protection due to the similar nature of the two pox viruses.

Signs and symptoms of infection include fever, headache, muscle aches, backache, swollen lymph nodes, a general feeling of discomfort, and exhaustion. Within 1 to 3 days (sometimes longer) after the appearance of fever, the patient develops a papular rash. Death, when it occurs, is generally due to pneumonia.

So, you can easily infer that whatever is being projected and propagated about Monkeypox by the media has already been planned meticulously. So much so that when and how will the heading and titles of news articles be rolled out and when and which image to be used for which purpose, all the details have been pre-decided and planned.

The future planning discussed in the document is equally interesting. Page number 10 of the document is fascinating, where it mentions in detail from May and June 2022 till January 2023, the spread of Monkeypox and the number of countries it will spread across. The page also provides an account of how the vaccine will be rolled out in the market for the same.

Check the moves 1, 2 & 3 and round table given in the pic next and the dates mentioned against each MOVE. Visit **www.biswaroop.com/pandemichoax** to download this document.

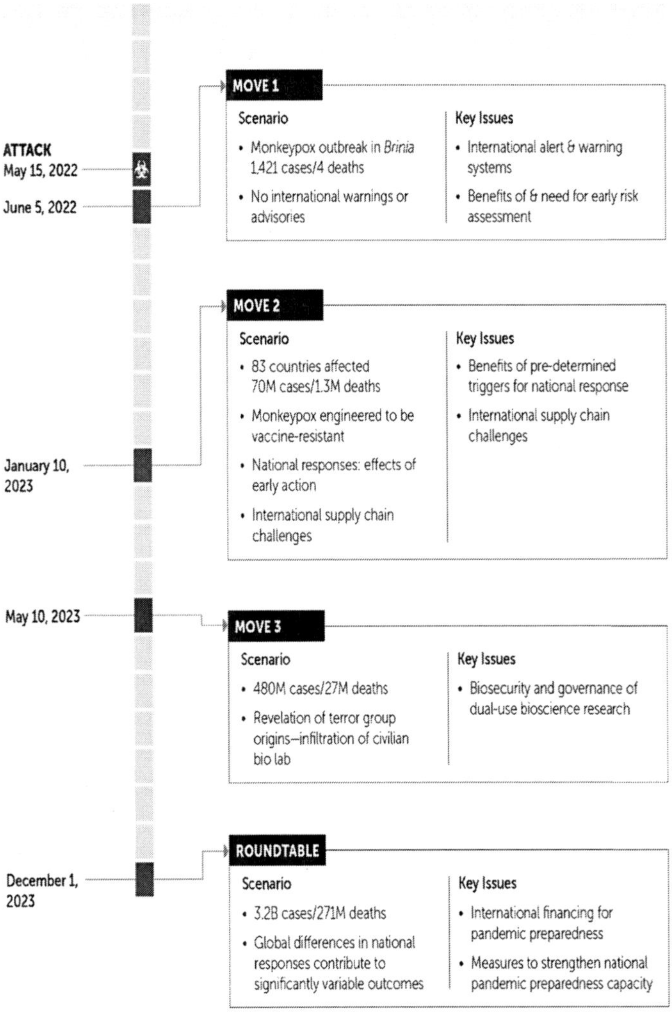
ATTACK
May 15, 2022
June 5, 2022
MOVE 1
Scenario
• Monkeypox outbreak in Brinia 1,421 cases/4 deaths
• No international warnings or advisories
Key Issues
• International alert & warning systems
• Benefits of & need for early risk assessment
January 10, 2023
MOVE 2
Scenario
• 83 countries affected 70M cases/1.3M deaths
• Monkeypox engineered to be vaccine-resistant
• National responses: effects of early action
• International supply chain challenges
Key Issues
• Benefits of pre-determined triggers for national response
• International supply chain challenges
May 10, 2023
MOVE 3
Scenario
• 480M cases/27M deaths
• Revelation of terror group origins—infiltration of civilian bio lab
Key Issues
• Biosecurity and governance of dual-use bioscience research
December 1, 2023
ROUNDTABLE
Scenario
• 3.2B cases/271M deaths
• Global differences in national responses contribute to significantly variable outcomes
Key Issues
• International financing for pandemic preparedness
• Measures to strengthen national pandemic preparedness capacity

Further, in details it states from the time duration from May 10, 2023 till December 1, 2023 the various stages of planning and execution.

So as you can see there is nothing to worry about as the comprehensive step-by-step planning pertaining to the spread of Monkeypox and its cure has already been laid out till December 2023.

Moving forward to page number 11, it is very interesting to note that it is established that those who comply with the directives of WHO will see a lower graph in terms of deaths rate while those who oppose or do not comply will be depicted by a much higher graph of death rate.

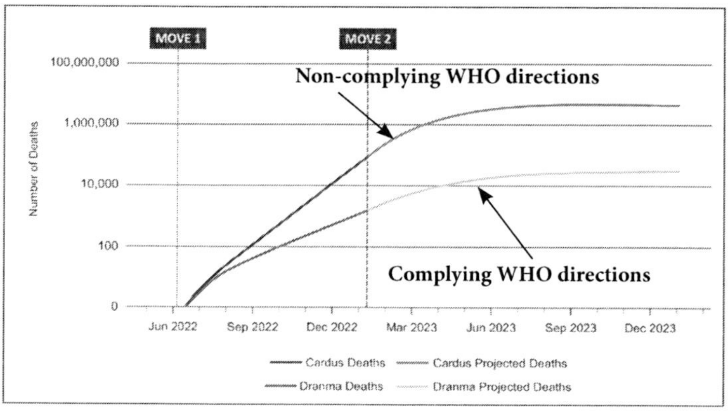

Death rates for complying & non complying WHO directions

While so far you have been able to understand the game of cases, let me explain it in detail now. Here take a look at a scary title called Case Fatality Rate (CFR) where it is assumed that 10% casualties of Monkeypox will for sure succumb to death.

Parameter	Symbol	Value	Source
Transmission rate	Beta (β)	0.175	scenario assumption
Pre-symptomatic period	–	8 days	[14]
Mild infection duration	–	14 days	[15]
Hospital stay (recovery/death)	–	18 days	ibid.
Asymptomatic cases	–	0%	[16]
Hospitalization rate	Rho1 (ρ_1)	50%	[17] and scenario assumption
ICU need for hospitalized	Rho2 (ρ_2)	40%	ibid.
Death for ICU cases	Mu (μ)	50%	ibid.
Total Case Fatality Rate (CFR)	–	10%	[18]

The details of this explanation are mentioned on page number 29. First random testing will be carried out on all those who become suspects of carriers of the virus. Anybody who travels through air or who visits hospital, can be identified as a suspect.

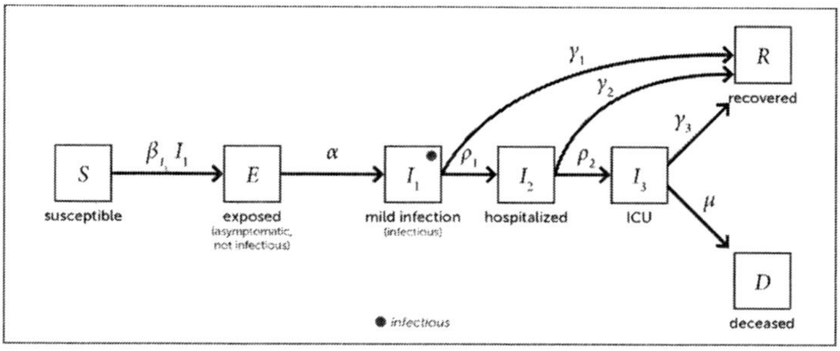

Flow chart for carrying out tests and future course of actions/procedure

In order to carry out random testing they have already devised a Kit as shown:

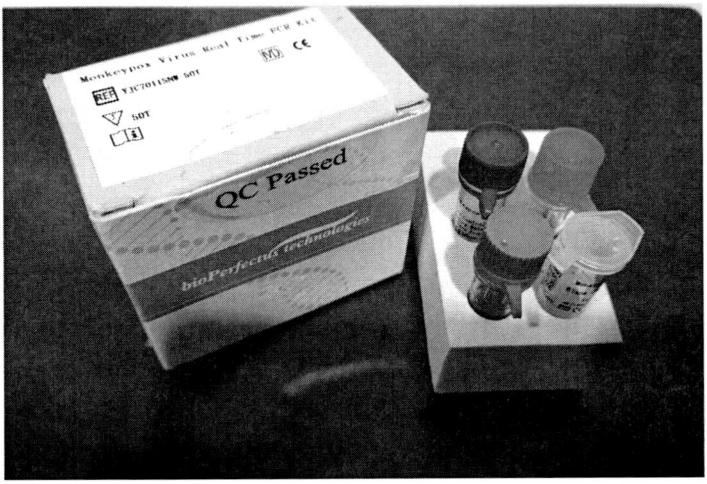

Monkeypox Virus RT-PCR Test Kit

bioPerfectus technologies

Certificate of Inspection
合格证

Product 品名：	Monkeypox Virus Real Time PCR kit 猴痘病毒核酸检测试剂盒（荧光PCR法）
Cat. No. 货号：	YJC70115NW-50T
Packaging 规格：	50tests/kit 50人份/盒
Inspector 检验员：	01
Lot No. 生产批号：	20220601
Manufacture Date (YYYY/MM/DD) 生产日期：	2022. 06. 01
Expiry Date (YYYY/MM/DD) 有效期：	2023. 05. 31

QC PASS

Jiangsu Bioperfectus Technologies Co., Ltd.
江苏硕世生物科技股份有限公司

3rd and 4th floors of Building A(G19), 4th floor of Building F(G14), Ground floor of Building G20, Shuaiyu Village, Fuye village, Sixiang town, Taizhou National Medical, Hi-tech Development Zone, 225300 Taizhou, Jiangsu, PEOPLE'S REPUBLIC OF CHINA.

泰州市开发区寺巷富野村、帅于村 A 幢（G19）第三层厂房与第三、第四层办研区，泰州市开发区寺巷富野村、帅于 村 F 幢（G14 四楼办研区），泰州市国家医药高新技术产业园寺巷富野村、帅于村（G20）

The cost of the kit is INR 1.5 lakh. If we look at it closely, we can see that it has been manufactured in China and is dated June 01, 2022.

The kit comprises a Positive Control, a Negative Control also known as Blank Control. Along with this we have a reactive test kit and a Detection mix. This is the complete kit to test for Monkeypox and costs INR 1.5 lakh. Using this kit, we were able to conduct 44 tests. In other words we were able to use this kit a total of 44 times.

We cleverly used a human sample, of Dr Namita Gupta. She took her own blood sample, tested it in an RT-PCR Test machine. RT-PCR (Reverse Transcription Polymerase Chain Reaction) Test is also known as the ultimate gold standard for testing.

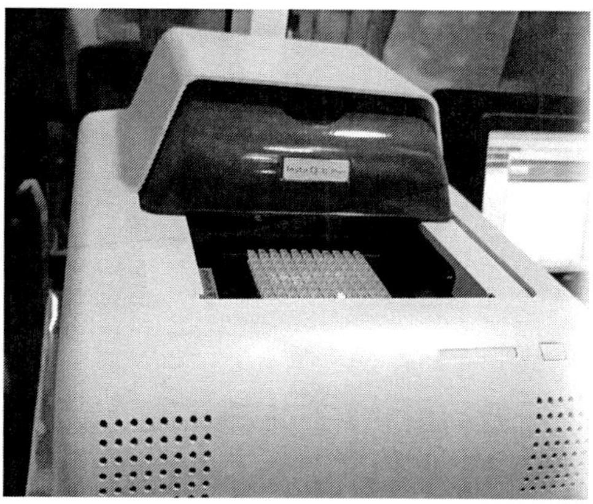

RT-PCR Test Machine

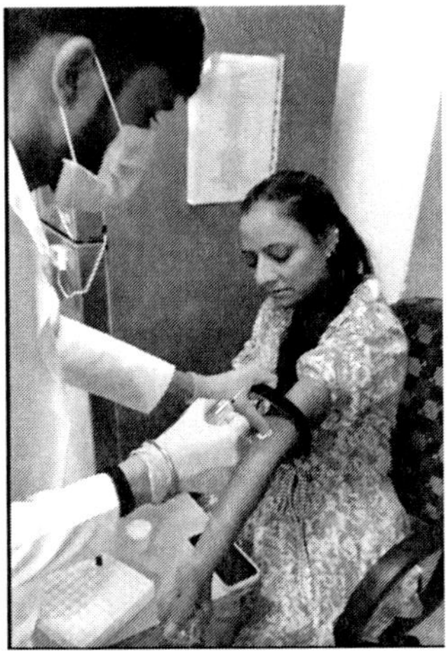

Dr. Namita Gupta blood sample for testing Monkeypox Virus

So, she gave her blood sample to be tested by this machine for Monkeypox. She gave the same blood sample several times for testing. This means she divided her blood sample into various parts and one-by-one gave them all to be tested for Monkeypox by the RT-PCR Machine.

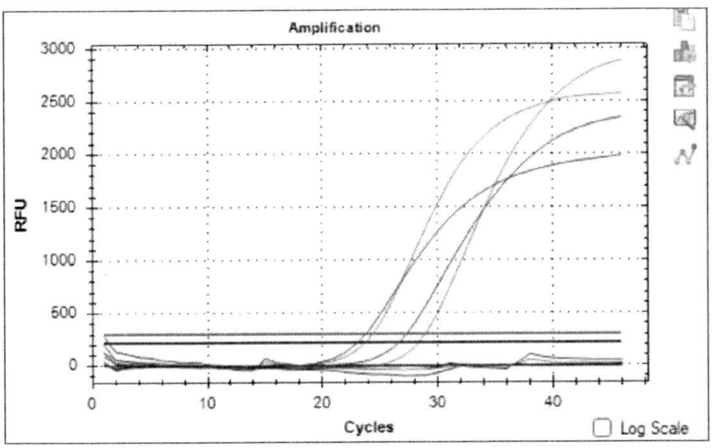

Figure-1

	1	2	3	4	5	6	7	8	9	10	11	12
A	Unk											
B	Unk											
C	Unk											
D	Unk											
E												
F	Neg											
G	Pos											
H												

Figure-2

Well	Fluor	Target	Content	Sample	Cq
A01	FAM		Unkn		N/A
B01	FAM		Unkn		N/A
C01	FAM		Unkn		N/A
D01	FAM		Unkn		26.65
F01	FAM		Neg Ctrl		N/A
G01	FAM		Pos Ctrl		23.11
A01	VIC		Unkn		N/A
B01	VIC		Unkn		N/A
C01	VIC		Unkn		N/A
D01	VIC		Unkn		28.94
F01	VIC		Neg Ctrl		N/A
G01	VIC		Pos Ctrl		24.35

Figure-3

As you can see in the table-3, the result of sample A01, the FAM (known to be Monkeypox gene indicator) is found N/A.

Similarly blood sample B01; C01 also tested negative for supposedly Monkeypox virus. However, the fourth test i.e D01, the sample of the same blood tested positive for Monkeypox with cycle threshold of 26.65.

Next, the F01 sample is a standard negative control and the G01, is the positive control showing cycle threshold as 23.11. So ultimately, on the basis of above test results, we can declare Dr. Namita as Monkeypox positive.

And for her, it was not an easy task to be diagnosed as Monkeypox positive; she worked very hard to prove herself Monkeypox positive. She got her blood sample tested for Monkeypox several times earlier the same day as well. However all these test came out to be Monkeypox negative (as can be seen from the table given on the next page).

28 JULY 2022 RUN MONKEY POX ..pcrd

07/28/2022 15:52

Report Information

User: BioRad/admin
Data File Name: 28 JULY 2022 RUN MONKEY POX ..pcrd
Data File Path: C:\Users\Bio-Rad\Desktop
Well Group Name: All Wells
Report Differs from Last Save: No

Run Setup

Run Information

Run Date: 07/28/2022 14:29
Run User: admin
Run Type: User-defined
Plate File: MONKEY POX TEMPLATE..pltd
ID:
Notes:
Sample Volume: 25
Temperature Control Mode: Calculated
Lid Temperature: 105
Base Serial Number: 795BR02679
Optical Head Serial Number: 795BR02679

Protocol

1: 95.0°C for 5:00
2: 95.0°C for 0:10
3: 58.0°C for 0:30
Plate Read
4: GOTO 2, 45 more times

Plate Display

	1	2	3	4	5	6	7	8	9	10	11	12
A	Unk FAM VIC	Unk FAM VIC	Unk FAM VIC	Unk FAM VIC	Unk FAM VIC	Unk FAM VIC						
B	Unk FAM VIC	Unk FAM VIC	Unk FAM VIC	Unk FAM VIC	Unk FAM VIC	Unk FAM VIC						
C	Unk FAM VIC	Unk FAM VIC	Unk FAM VIC	Unk FAM VIC	Unk FAM VIC	NTC FAM VIC						
D	Unk FAM VIC	Unk FAM VIC	Unk FAM VIC	Unk FAM VIC	Unk FAM VIC	Pos FAM VIC						
E	Unk FAM VIC	Unk FAM VIC	Unk FAM VIC	Unk FAM VIC	Unk FAM VIC							
F	Unk FAM VIC	Unk FAM VIC	Unk FAM VIC	Unk FAM VIC	Unk FAM VIC							

Plate Display

	1	2	3	4	5	6	7	8	9	10	11	12
G	Unk FAM VIC	Unk FAM VIC	Unk FAM VIC	Unk FAM VIC	Unk FAM VIC							
H	Unk FAM VIC	Unk FAM VIC	Unk FAM VIC	Unk FAM VIC	Unk FAM VIC							

Quantification

Step #: 3
Analysis Mode: Fluorophore
Cq Determination: Single Threshold
Baseline Method:
FAM: Auto Calculated
VIC: Auto Calculated
Threshold Setting:
FAM: 106.56, User Defined
VIC: 86.01, User Defined

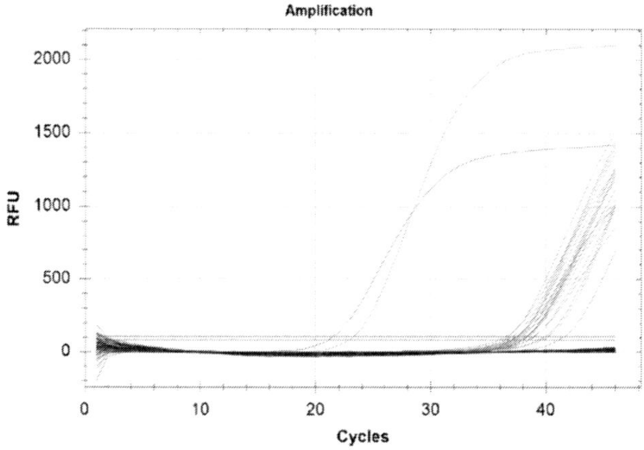

Quantification Data

Well	Fluor	Target	Content	Sample	Cq	Cq Mean	Cq Std. Dev
A01	FAM		Unkn		N/A	0.00	0.000
A02	FAM		Unkn		N/A	0.00	0.000
A03	FAM		Unkn		N/A	0.00	0.000
A04	FAM		Unkn		N/A	0.00	0.000
A05	FAM		Unkn		N/A	0.00	0.000
A06	FAM		Unkn		N/A	0.00	0.000
B01	FAM		Unkn		N/A	0.00	0.000
B02	FAM		Unkn		N/A	0.00	0.000
B03	FAM		Unkn		N/A	0.00	0.000
B04	FAM		Unkn		N/A	0.00	0.000

Quantification Data

Well	Fluor	Target	Content	Sample	Cq	Cq Mean	Cq Std. Dev
B05	FAM		Unkn		N/A	0.00	0.000
B06	FAM		Unkn		N/A	0.00	0.000
C01	FAM		Unkn		N/A	0.00	0.000
C02	FAM		Unkn		N/A	0.00	0.000
C03	FAM		Unkn		N/A	0.00	0.000
C04	FAM		Unkn		N/A	0.00	0.000
C05	FAM		Unkn		N/A	0.00	0.000
C06	FAM		NTC		N/A	0.00	0.000
D01	FAM		Unkn		N/A	0.00	0.000
D02	FAM		Unkn		N/A	0.00	0.000
D03	FAM		Unkn		N/A	0.00	0.000
D04	FAM		Unkn		N/A	0.00	0.000
D05	FAM		Unkn		N/A	0.00	0.000
D06	FAM		Pos Ctrl		21.46	21.46	0.000
E01	FAM		Unkn		N/A	0.00	0.000
E02	FAM		Unkn		N/A	0.00	0.000
E03	FAM		Unkn		N/A	0.00	0.000

Well	Fluor	Target	Content	Sample	Cq	Cq Mean	Cq Std. Dev
E04	FAM		Unkn		N/A	0.00	0.000
E05	FAM		Unkn		N/A	0.00	0.000
F01	FAM		Unkn		N/A	0.00	0.000
F02	FAM		Unkn		N/A	0.00	0.000
F03	FAM		Unkn		N/A	0.00	0.000
F04	FAM		Unkn		N/A	0.00	0.000
F05	FAM		Unkn		N/A	0.00	0.000
G01	FAM		Unkn		N/A	0.00	0.000
G02	FAM		Unkn		N/A	0.00	0.000
G03	FAM		Unkn		N/A	0.00	0.000
G04	FAM		Unkn		N/A	0.00	0.000
G05	FAM		Unkn		N/A	0.00	0.000
H01	FAM		Unkn		N/A	0.00	0.000
H02	FAM		Unkn		N/A	0.00	0.000
H03	FAM		Unkn		N/A	0.00	0.000
H04	FAM		Unkn		N/A	0.00	0.000
H05	FAM		Unkn		N/A	0.00	0.000

The tests you see above are the tests that were conducted many times over. However, Dr Namita did not lose hope. After testing her blood sample many times in the RT-PCR machine, she was finally rewarded and became the world's first Monkeypox virus positive doctor.

If you also have the desire to be rewarded with titles such as the World's first Monkeypox Engineer, World's first Monkeypox Chartered Accountant etc., all you need is a little bit of money and a testing lab close by. Simply visit the lab and give your blood sample to be tested by the RT-PCR machine many times over. After giving your blood sample to be tested 10, 15, 20, or even 25 times, chances are that you too will definitely be diagnosed as Monkeypox positive at least once.

This is how this game is being played with human lives wherein any individual can be considered Monkeypox positive with the only condition that he must get his blood sample tested repeatedly. It can therefore, be understood that in the newspaper **'The Hindu' dated July 29, 2022**

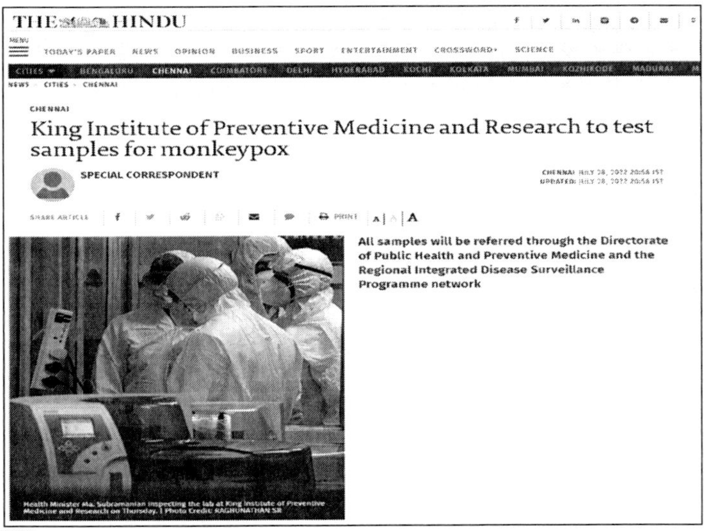

THE HINDU

TODAY'S PAPER NEWS OPINION BUSINESS SPORT ENTERTAINMENT CROSSWORD+ SCIENCE

CITIES BENGALURU CHENNAI COIMBATORE DELHI HYDERABAD KOCHI KOLKATA MUMBAI KOZHIKODE MADURAI

NEWS › CITIES › CHENNAI

CHENNAI

King Institute of Preventive Medicine and Research to test samples for monkeypox

SPECIAL CORRESPONDENT

CHENNAI JULY 28, 2022 20:58 IST
UPDATED: JULY 28, 2022 20:58 IST

SHARE ARTICLE PRINT A A

Health Minister Ma. Subramanian inspecting the lab at King Institute of Preventive Medicine and Research on Thursday. | Photo Credit: RAGHUNATHAN SR

All samples will be referred through the Directorate of Public Health and Preventive Medicine and the Regional Integrated Disease Surveillance Programme network where it has been written that provisions for mass testing have already begun for times to come. So it is obvious that lakhs of people will undergo testing for Monkeypox. As per our experience, when 10 lakh individuals will be tested for Monkeypox, around one lakh individuals will automatically be detected as positive. Given the design of this game, the testing mechanisms and facilities, it goes without saying that when anyone is tested repeatedly for a few times, he will be declared Monkey-pox positive at least once for sure.

All these tests will be conducted randomly, as a part of the suspicion. Such positive cases will then be declared as asymptomatic. The next step in the process is mentioned to be 'Asymptomatic Exposed', which will then need to be converted into the category of Mild Infection. For this purpose the entire paraphernalia of medications will come into play. **TPoxx** has recently been approved by the FDA.

This TPoxx in reality is a dangerous medication which can be instrumental in any person's demise. When enquired about the clinical trials conducted towards approving TPoxx, the FDA responds with a negative reply. The FDA has no data that can prove that this medication will benefit human health, and how it will impact in curing the so-called Monkeypox. Even if there exists such an illness in reality, then they have no data to support how this specific medication cures an individual of it. In fact, a point to be noted here is that they can't have any support data as they don't have any patients either. The FDA went ahead and simply approved TPoxx despite a lack of supporting data. Whenever we see a tag mentioning FDA approved, we think that an array of tests and precautions must be in place for something to be approved by FDA. But here the FDA themselves are claiming

FDA U.S. FOOD & DRUG
ADMINISTRATION

Monkeypox Fast Facts

TPOXX (tecovirimat)

If you have monkeypox symptoms, talk to your healthcare provider even if you haven't had contact with someone who has monkeypox.

What you need to know:

- **TPOXX is an antiviral drug approved by the FDA in 2018 to treat smallpox in adults and children.**
- **There are no FDA-approved or authorized treatment for monkeypox virus infections,** and no data establishing the safety or effectiveness of using TPOXX to treat monkeypox in humans.
- TPOXX may be used **for people with severe disease or who are more likely to get severely ill,** like patients with weakened immune systems.

About the drug:

- The FDA approved TPOXX for smallpox under the FDA's Animal Rule regulations, which allows for approval of certain drugs and biological products when human efficacy studies are not ethical and field trials to study the effectiveness of drugs or biological products are not feasible.
- Human efficacy studies of smallpox disease are not feasible because smallpox has been eradicated globally and exposing people to smallpox virus for the purpose of a clinical trial is not ethical. Due to scientific and logistical limitations with the use of smallpox virus in animal models, the efficacy of TPOXX was established in animal models using related viruses, specifically non-human primates infected with monkeypox virus and rabbits infected with rabbitpox virus. These studies demonstrated improved survival in animals that received TPOXX compared to animals that received placebo.
- There are currently no data demonstrating the effectiveness of TPOXX for the treatment of smallpox or monkeypox in humans. TPOXX has only been tested in healthy human volunteers, without smallpox or monkeypox infection, to assess safety.
- Drugs that are effective in animal studies are not always effective in humans. Conducting randomized, controlled trials to assess TPOXX's safety and efficacy in humans with monkeypox infections is essential.
- As monkeypox was endemic in other parts of the world (e.g., the Democratic Republic of Congo), it was not eligible for approval for the treatment of monkeypox disease under the FDA's Animal Rule regulations because it was both ethical and feasible to conduct clinical trials in humans.
- The prescribing information contains more information about the drug.

that they have no data to prove the reason for the approval of TPoxx.

Let us dig further into the history of this medicine.

We know that with the effective use of the media and newspaper, a common man by now, has been educated about the symptoms to recognize Monkeypox which includes headache, fever, weakness, body ache and rashes on the skin/body. And if you happen to have some or all of these symptoms then you can conclude that you are a potential patient of Monkeypox and likely to be given Tpoxx medicine as a cure for it.

If we look at the general side-effects of the medicine TPoxx, we see that patients who take this medicine are liable to experience headache, fever, weakness, body ache, and rashes on the body. So the side-effects of TPoxx are the same as the declared symptoms of Monkeypox.

Media Promoted Symptoms of Monkeypox	**Clinically Proven Side effects of Tpoxx**
Headache	Headache
Fever	Fever
Weakness	Weakness
Body ache	Body ache
Rashes on the skin	Rashes on the skin

In other words, first a healthy individual is declared through the test that he is Monkeypox positive, then he will be given TPoxx and due to the side effects of this drug, when all those symptoms will start to emerge (they will say), "Look! you have all the symptoms of Monkeypox". In the next step, the dosage of the medication will be increased, and then it is possible that some of the people may not be able to withstand the side effect and even die. And those who will manage to recover despite all, but due to side-effects of these medicines, they will remain unwell throughout their life.

This is exactly similar to the case where crores of people who made the mistake and went to the hospital to seek treatment for Covid-19 but by God's grace, are still alives, you must have noticed that some of them are suffering from diabetes or arthritis or kidney diseases or even weakness. It is common to find them struggling with some disease or another throughout their life. So the game that has been played is that permanently you are going to be sick.

When we move forward, what I found most fear-striking is the fact that the preparation for 2023 is that they already have a full-planning of a lockdown. While we are still struggling to get back on track, after the (2020-2021) lockdown was lifted, however, there is an impending lockdown looming all

Document from NTI, page-31

Strengthening Global Systems to Prevent and Respond to High-Consequence Biological Threats

and leaves the R well above 1. The "Moderate" response countries open up in January, increasing R to approximately 2.2, before locking down in the summer of 2023 when the outbreak is undeniable. Finally, the "Effective" response countries lock down aggressively in February 2023 and keep R below 1 throughout the remainder of the exercise.

The combined global pandemic leads to more than three billion cumulative cases and more than 270 million deaths by the end of December 2023. At the peak of the pandemic, nearly 500 million individuals are infected at the same time, and there are 161 million people simultaneously in need of hospitalization.

The model was written in Python, with configuration and visualization through Jupyter notebooks.

over again in 2023. So you must start planning and preparing for your future bread and butter with lockdown in mind just like I have already planned my future.

I have taken a cart which consists of Monkeypox bags and T-shirts. I feel monkeys will be in fashion very soon so there will be a Monkeypox bag. It's a hardy bag. If you want, we can customise this bag for you and we will remove the monkey photo and use your photo on this bag. If you are already set to be fooled by the Monkeypox pandemic, why not put your own photo on this bag. So you have this bag & this T-Shirt which can be bought from my 'thela/cart' @ www.biswaroop.com/shop. It is ready for sale. So you also make preparations, because this time it may be 'You' who becomes jobless & homeless in the same way as it happened with millions of labourers during the last forced lockdown.

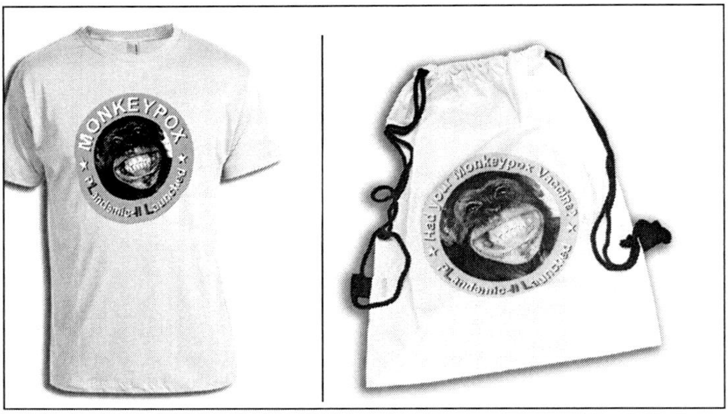

What I mean to say is that planning is already done. Now, you will think, this is a "Plandemic," there is no real disease as such, so this means there is no need to panic or no need to feel the danger of this so-called risked disease. That is true that there is no danger from the so-called Monkeypox as such, but there is no other 'absolute danger' – we still cannot claim that yet. This is because, as per our observation and what we have seen on those patients who visit our hospitals, (HIIMS-hospital) all those who are vaccinated have experienced certain rashes post vaccine. As a result of the vaccine, the body has experienced a variety of eruptions on the skin, as a side–effect of Covid-19 vaccine.

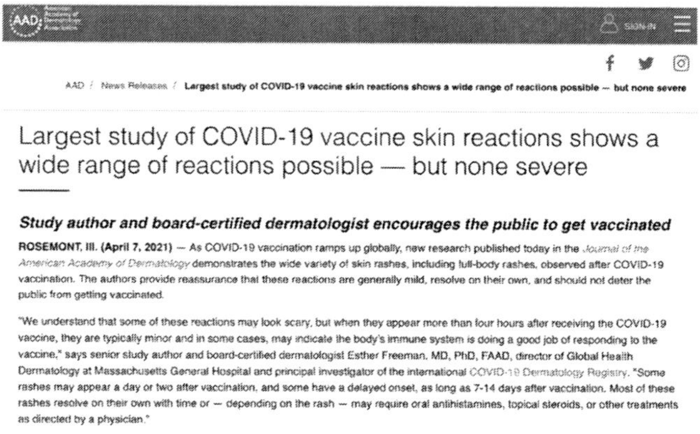

AAD / News Releases / Largest study of COVID-19 vaccine skin reactions shows a wide range of reactions possible — but none severe

Largest study of COVID-19 vaccine skin reactions shows a wide range of reactions possible — but none severe

Study author and board-certified dermatologist encourages the public to get vaccinated

ROSEMONT, Ill. (April 7, 2021) — As COVID-19 vaccination ramps up globally, new research published today in the *Journal of the American Academy of Dermatology* demonstrates the wide variety of skin rashes, including full-body rashes, observed after COVID-19 vaccination. The authors provide reassurance that these reactions are generally mild, resolve on their own, and should not deter the public from getting vaccinated.

"We understand that some of these reactions may look scary, but when they appear more than four hours after receiving the COVID-19 vaccine, they are typically minor and in some cases, may indicate the body's immune system is doing a good job of responding to the vaccine," says senior study author and board-certified dermatologist Esther Freeman, MD, PhD, FAAD, director of Global Health Dermatology at Massachusetts General Hospital and principal investigator of the international COVID-19 Dermatology Registry. "Some rashes may appear a day or two after vaccination, and some have a delayed onset, as long as 7-14 days after vaccination. Most of these rashes resolve on their own with time or — depending on the rash — may require oral antihistamines, topical steroids, or other treatments as directed by a physician."

Now, the game that they are going to play is that whatever skin maladies or eruptions are there on the skin, all these side-effects will now be termed Monkeypox. This means they are aiming and covering two points from a single shot of arrow. So on the one hand they are saved from acknowledging that these are possible side-effects of the vaccine and on the other hand, they have found a ready platform to start the new game of Monkeypox.

Now there must be two probable questions on your mind – first question – God forbid that you get any kind of eruption on your body, or you start getting a physical symptom, or you start getting a skin disease, so in that case what will you do?

Your second question could be that this game that has started might result in a possible pandemic or a lockdown. What should we do in such a condition?

And the answer to the first question i.e. what should you do if you start getting physical symptoms like fever, body ache, headache or skin eruptions, is to follow- 'Skin Detox Method'.

Skin Detox Method (SDM)

SDM = Heat Protocol + 3 Step Flu Diet + Decoction / Bath Therapy

STEP 1

When you observe the first sign of Flu such as cold, cough, fever or fatigue, you should take Lower Leg Hot Water

With 1st sign of Flu / 1st 30 min

STEP-I

Lower leg hot water immersion (42°C to 43°C)

With lavender oil

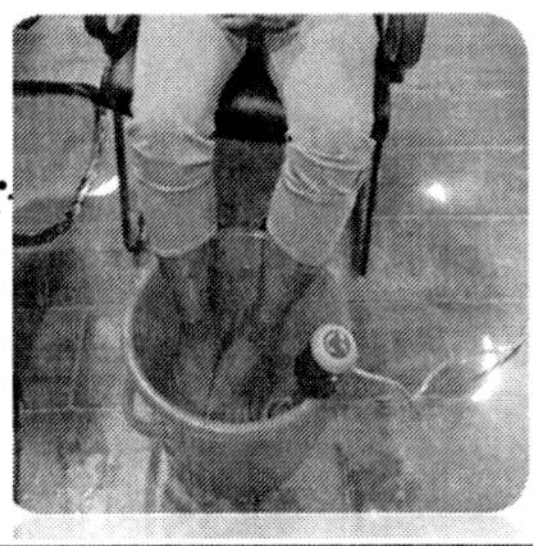

Babar Ali et al. Essential oils used in aromatherapy, A systemic review: July 2015 Asian Pacific Journal of Tropical Biomedicine 5(8):589-598

3 Step Heat Protocol

Immersion (LLHWI) therapy i.e. take hot water (approx. 42 degrees to 43 degrees) in a bucket.

Add one tablespoon of Lavender oil in it. Dip your legs in the bucket. The aroma of Lavender oil de-stresses the patient and hot water cures the Flu effect. This therapy should be performed for about 30 minutes and while the legs are placed inside the bucket, the temperature of water should be maintained between 42-43 degrees. To maintain the temperature, keep another bucket full of water having temperature more than 50^{0}C; remove two mugs of water from the bucket in which the legs are dipped and add two mugs of water from the other bucket. If you repeat the process after every 5 minutes, it will ensure that the temperature of water is maintained to 42-43 degrees throughout the duration of the first step. To make the LLHWI therapy more effective, you can put a blanket on the patient.

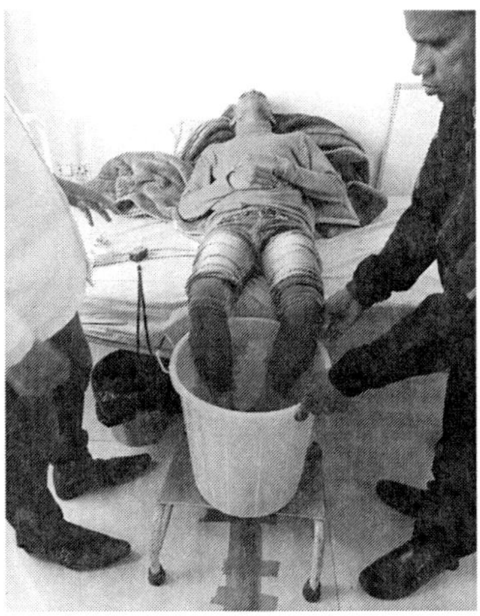

If the patient is too weak to sit down (since this therapy is best done while sitting), make him lie down and dip both his feet in the hot water bucket as shown in the picture. In this case, the patient may forgo step 2 and step 3.

STEP 2

Take 500 ml hot water (whose temperature is approx. > 80°C). Squeeze one lemon (juice) in it. Start sipping it slowly. In this manner, we are providing heat and humidity through the nose and mouth, which helps in destroying the virus in its early stage.

With 1st sign of Flu / 1st 30 min

STEP-II

Sipping very-very hot water(>80°C) about 500 ml with lemon juice drops

3 Step Heat Protocol

STEP 3

The third step is nasal irrigation commonly known as Jal Neti (one of the famous techniques mentioned in Ayurveda).

Take 200 ml hot water (approx. 40°C - 42°C). Add one spoon of salt in it and perform Jal Neti as described in the Ayurveda. This procedure needs expertise.

With 1st sign of Flu / 1st 30 min

STEP-III

Nasal irrigation (Jal Neti)(40°C to 42°C) about 200 ml with salt (one spoon)

3 Step Heat Protocol

To perform it in a simple manner, take a squeezy bottle (like tomato sauce plastic bottle) and perform Jal Neti for around 2-3 minutes. This step can also be done simultaneously with the first step.

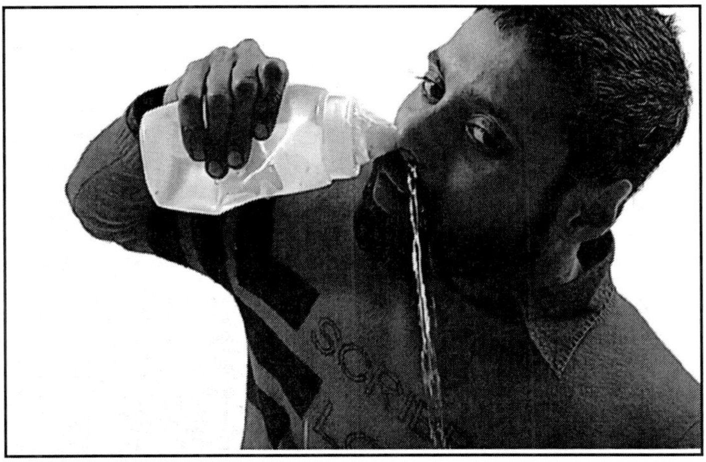

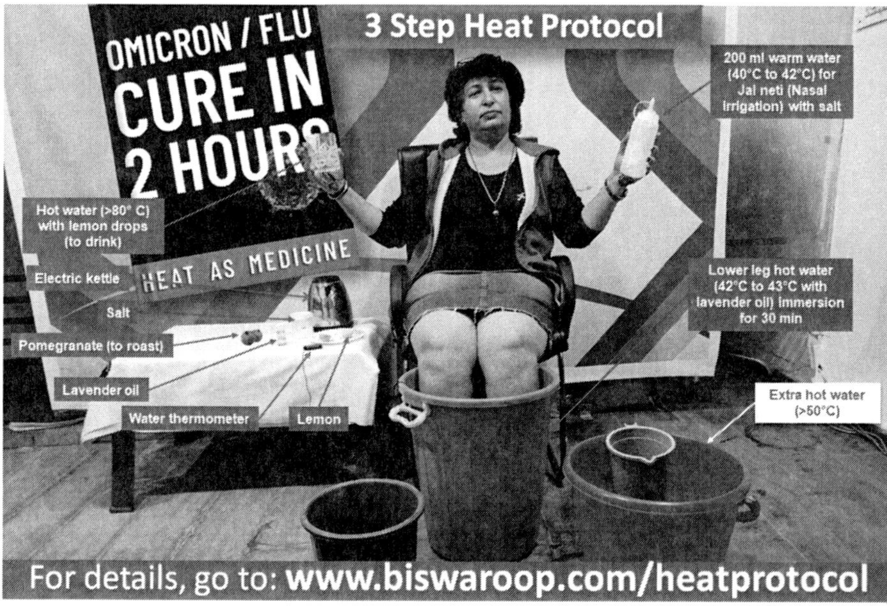
OMICRON / FLU
CURE IN
2 HOUR
3 Step Heat Protocol
200 ml warm water (40°C to 42°C) for Jal neti (Nasal irrigation) with salt
Hot water (>80° C) with lemon drops (to drink)
HEAT AS MEDICINE
Electric kettle
Salt
Pomegranate (to roast)
Lavender oil
Water thermometer
Lemon
Lower leg hot water (42°C to 43°C with lavender oil) immersion for 30 min
Extra hot water (>50°C)
For details, go to: www.biswaroop.com/heatprotocol

It is advised that by repeating the above three steps 2-3 times would provide relief from Flu. The three step heat protocol is depicted in brief:

3 Step Heat Protocol – 30 min	
Step I →	**LL HWI (Lavender oil)**
Step II→	**Sipping very hot water (500 ml + Lemon)**
Step III→	**Jal Neti (200 ml water + salt)**

It is also suggested that even after getting well, follow the three step Flu diet for 3 days.

3 STEP FLU DIET

Day 1 (Liquid)

$\frac{\text{Weight of patient (kg)}}{10}$ (glasses of fresh Citrus fruit juice)

+

$\frac{\text{Weight (kg)}}{10}$ (glasses of coconut water)

3 STEP FLU DIET

Day 2 (Fluid)

$\frac{\text{Weight}}{20}$ (glasses of Citrus fruit juice)

+

$\frac{\text{Weight}}{20}$ (glasses of coconut water)

+

Weight x 5 (gm of Tomato+Cucumber)

3 STEP FLU DIET

Day 3 (Solid)

$\frac{\text{Weight}}{30}$	(glasses of Citrus fruit juice) + $\frac{\text{Weight}}{30}$ (glasses of coconut water)	**Breakfast**
Weight x 5	(gm of Tomato +Cucumber)	**Lunch**
Normal home cooked food		**Dinner**

Decoction/Bath Therapy:

STEP 1: Morning Kadha/ Decoction- Drink Amla Juice (Indian Gooseberry Juice) in the Morning: A 60 kg person should take 60 ml amla juice/ Indian gooseberry juice in 60 ml of water and sip it.

STEP 2: Evening Kadha/ Decoction- Neem Kadha : Boil 10-12 Neem leaves in 200 ml water and condense to half i.e. 100 ml. Sieve it and sip this kadha.

STEP 3: Neem Bath: Take half kg neem leaves along with twigs and put it in a bucket of water and keep it overnight. This neem water can be used for bathing in the morning after removing twigs and leaves.

In-case you forgot to soak neem leaves in water, you can take half kg of neem leaves with twigs in 2 litres of water and boil it till it reduces to half the quantity. After removing the leaves and twins, put this medicated water in the bucket full of water and bathe.

The answer to your second question i.e., this game that has started might result in a possible pandemic or a lockdown. What should we do in such a situation? So what you can do is to create awareness among people and bring out the truth. A simple way to do it, can be through this evidence based book in your hand. Distribute and spread this book/e-book to as many people as you can. Translate it into as many languages as you can and spread it like wildfire. Because the evidences given in this book will help people in understanding the facts and truth about Monkeypox and once they understand the truth they will not be scared and will neither go for the test nor take any vaccine. And when people will unite and raise their voice against vaccines, their unity and strength will bring an end to this 'Plandemic' and the deathly game. To read the e-book visit the link: **www.biswaroop.com/pandemichoax**

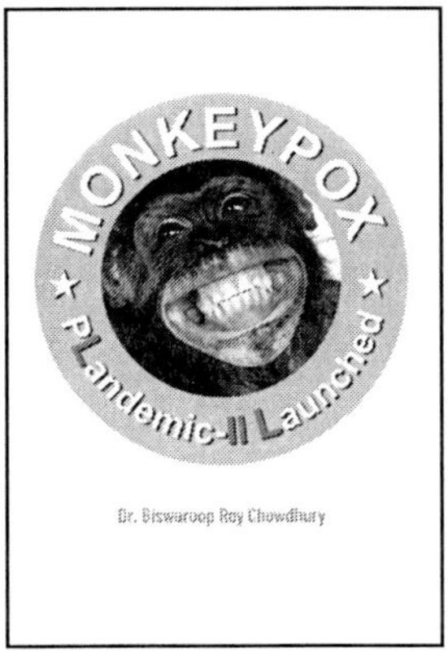

To read complete articles/references/documents mentioned in the book visit the link: **www.biswaroop.com/pandemichoax**

Pseudo Illness

Illness can be categorised into two types; one is an actual illness wherein the person is experiencing discomfort in the body like headache, vomiting, body ache, weakness, depression and more. The second category is a pseudo illness, wherein you are made to believe that you are ill or will fall ill.

As discussed in the previous chapter and proven as well that in the case of Covid-19, people were not actually ill, (or just suffering from seasonal flu) they all opted for mass testing, and if the results were positive, they were lavelled as asymptomatic. Since they are declared patients of Covid-19, they were administered poisonous medicines like Remdesivir. Now, they actually become ill, not because of any pathogen or virus but because of the medicine and the treatment protocol

What we need to realise and think about here is that if a healthy person is lavelled as a patient it becomes a psychological burden. Furthermore keeping the person quarantined and treating them like an untouchable adds to the woes and that makes a lot of changes in the immune system and reduces immunity and the person becomes more prone to illness.

This journey from pseudo to real illness is what is happening in reality.

This not only occurred for Covid-19 but also planned for Monkeypox as you can witness. The mass testing preparation is carried on in the Airport. It is random testing and by fluke, anyone can come up positive. It is no real disease.

As discussed in the previous chapter the RT- PCR test kit (image), can fool anybody.

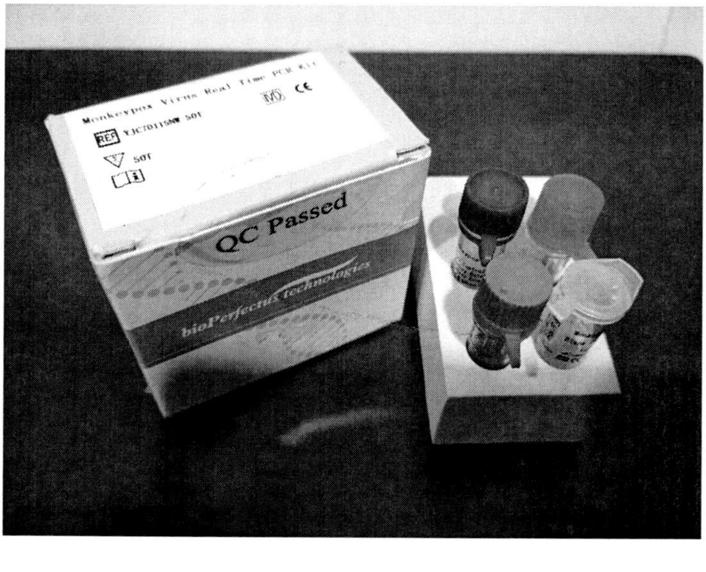

As a result of this test kit, people are being declared Monkeypox positive.

And now all unproven WHO protocols will be applicable and as a result of these protocols, a person can fall severely ill.

This practice of pseudo illness is not new; it has been adhered to for the last several decades.

As you see in the chart below :

WHO	1999	120/80
NIH	2003	120/80
European Guidelines	2003	140/90
Cochrane	2012	160/100
JNC-8	2014	150/90(<60yrs) 140/90 (>60yrs)

The blood pressure threshold for different organisations varies. The Cochrane which is a very reliable organisation, with the help of meta-analysis, if the BP is less than 160/100, then there is no need to control it.

If one administers drug to control it will cause more harm than good. Whereas WHO says if it's more than 120/80, it needs to be controlled by drugs.

So you see there are different organisations with various thresholds. So it is more likely that commercially established private hospitals and doctors would adhere to WHO protocol to mint more money from the patients. By doing so, they expand their base of patients. This means a per-son who is not a patient and has no illness and the BP monitor shows 130/90, he/she will be made to believe that they are a hypertensive patient and will be offered medications.

And this drug needs to be taken lifelong and the person now truly becomes a hypertension patient. The same thing can be seen for other parameters as well, like cholesterol.

As you can see in the diagram below,

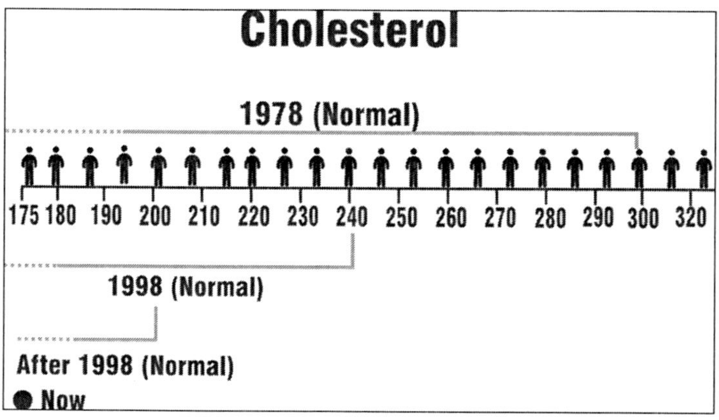

Untill 1978 according to Harrison's Principle of Internal Medicine book (the Bible of allopathic medicine), cholesterol of more than 300 was considered high cholesterol.

From 1998 onwards, that threshold was reduced to 240. So people whose cholesterol level was between 240 to 300 would be detected as having high cholesterol. And in the current scenario, the threshold is reduced to 200. So anyone above the range of 200 will be termed a high cholesterol patient.

And as you can see in the diagram (previous page), people whose cholesterol ranged between 200-300 were normal previously without any risks are now converted into high cholesterol patients.

Even if no symptoms or discomfort exist and no real illness, they are made to believe that they are ill and forced to consume medications like Statins.

Statins themselves cause a lot of harm to all organs and results in heart disease. And once you are diagnosed with heart disease, that means you migrated from a pseudo patient to a real patient.

Now let's see the story behind the thyroid.

Till 2003	TSH Range 0.1 to 6.0
Now	0.3 to 3.0

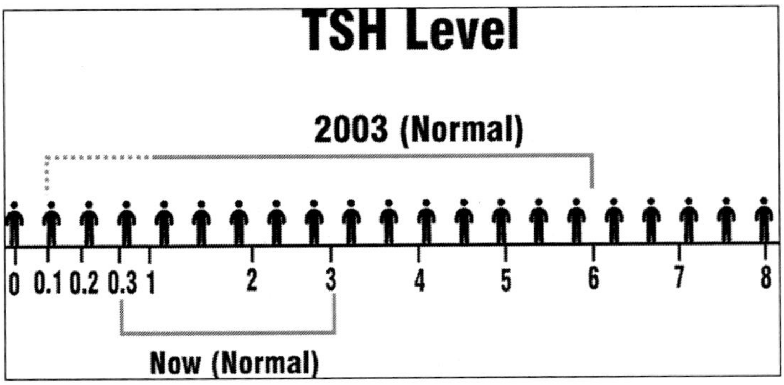

As you see from the chart, till 2003 if the range for TSH lay between 0.1 to 6.0 then the person had no thyroid issue. But now, the threshold has been drastically reduced to 0.3 to 3.0. For example, someone detected with TSH 4.0 will be put under medication and will be counselled to believe that one has to be dependent on medicine for the rest of their life.

And how these medicines affect people is important to understand. And once you start taking the medication, the dosage will keep increasing and it will also attract other ailments that affect the body's homeostasis (the central unifying concept of physiology and is defined as a self-regulating process by which an organism can maintain internal stability while adjusting to changing external conditions).

And further, you will be given more medications to control the complications arising due to thyroid medications.

Hence, it was a pseudo illness, but you are made to believe that you are a real patient.

As here, in the graph (previous page) above, you can see that till 2003, people from 3-6 fell under the normal category but now they are considered as patients.

Whether it is thyroid, cholesterol, BP or blood sugar, the history and the story remain the same.

Let's now talk about blood sugar. As long as your blood sugar is less than 250 mg/dl, according to the new ACP guidelines released in 2018, one doesn't have diabetes.

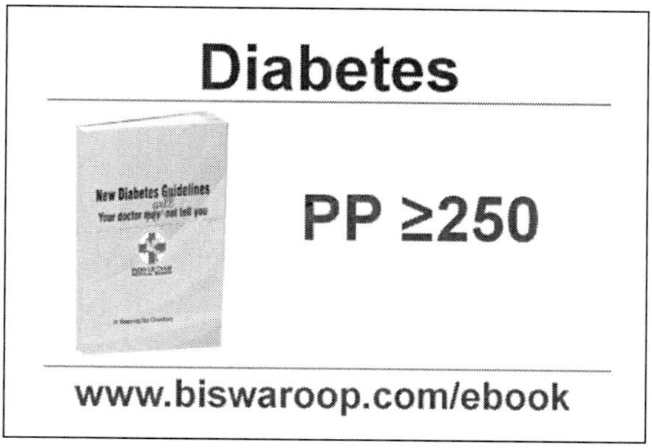

And this guideline is based on all the randomised controlled trials as shown below

Guidelines
ACP (2018) **ACCORD (2008)** **ADVANCE (2008)** **UKPDS-33 (1998)** **UKPDS-34 (1998)** **VADT (2015)**

All these randomised controlled trials conclude that if the blood sugar is less than 250 mg/dL and even then a patient is administered medicines, it will cause harm to the body.

As evidence suggests, if the blood sugar level is less than 250 mg/dL, then it's not required to be controlled or lowered further. If you still visit a doctor and your fasting blood sugar lies in the range of 120 mg/dL-130 mg/dL, you will be labelled as a pre-diabetic and would be prescribed medicines. And if you read all the trials, you will conclude that diabetes medicines themselves cause diabetes.

Hence, now you understand the difference between real and pseudo illness. Healthy people are made to believe that they are ill with the help of dubious diagnostic tests.

And now it is taken to the next level in the name of Monkeypox. As mass testing has already begun, now you needn't visit a doctor to become a pseudo patient.

If you are an Indian citizen and travelling via flight you will be randomly picked up at the airport for RT-PCR testing. If you are not lucky enough and you get diagnosed as Monkeypox positive; even though you might not have any symptoms, you will fall prey to these tactics and will be forced to consume unnecessary (any poisonous) medications. As a result, you turn from a pseudo patient to a real patient.

Let's take yet another example i.e. fever. We need to understand that fever is not an illness but a tool /mechanism for the body to fight the virus and bacteria. So, if you have fever do not suppress it with any medication.

In the last 80 years, all the trials conducted on fever (please refer to the table in th next page), have been listed here.

S.NO	Year	Reference
1	1942	"Fever in Ectotherms"; H. V. Ellingson and P. F. Clark, "The Influence of Artificial Fever on Mechanisms of Resistance," Journal of Immunology 43 (1942): 65-83; A. Lwoff
2	1959	"Factors Influencing the Evolution of Viral Diseases at the Cellular Level and the Organism," Bacterial Reviews 23 (1959): 109–24; D. Rodbard
3	1977	"Survival Value of Fever in Fish," Nature 267 (1977): 43–45; Kluger
4	1981	The Role of Regional Body Temperature in the Pathogenesis of Disease," New England Journal of Medicine 305 (1981): 808–14; E. Atkin
5	1983	"Treatment of Fever," New England Journal of Medicine 309 (1983): 925.
6	1992	animals... treated or not treated with antipyretics: M. J. Kluger, "Fever Revisited," Paediatrics 90 (1992): 720-24; J. B. Covert and W. W. Reynolds

Year	**Place**	Outcome(Placebo vs Paracetamol/Antipyretics)
1975	University of Illinois	Among the experimentally infected cold virus subjects, those treated with antipyretics, shed virus from their nose significantly longer.
1989	Johns Hopkins Hospital	Among the chickenpox patients, those given paracetamol, took significantly longer to heal
1990	University of Adelaide, South Australia	Among the experimentally infected rhinovirus volunteers, those given antipyretic had worse congestion, running nose, sneezing, sore throat and cough.
1994	Fujimoto Children's Hospital, Japan	Among the children with viral infection, those who received paracetamol were more likely to develop severe pneumonia requiring hospitalisation
2000	University of Maryland School of Medicine	Among the experimentally infected influenza virus volunteers, those who were treated with antipyretics had more severe illness and lasted 3 to 4 days longer

Year	Place	Outcome(Placebo vs Paracetamol/Antipyretics)
2005	University of Miami School of Medicine	Among the trauma patients, those who were given antipyretics to reduce fever were more likely to develop infection and more likely to die.
2019	Phramong kutklao College of Medicine	Among the dengue patients, those given paracetamol developed severe injury including haemorrhaged and acute kidney injury

And all the trials conclude that if you suffer from fever and consume Paracetamol to suppress the temperature, then it does severe damage and leads to a prolonged period of illness and suffering.

The obvious question that arises is when we suffer from fever, what should we do?

First, let's address what we should not do. Refrain from consuming medicines specifically, Paracetamol. According to Davidson's Principle and Practice of Medicine (23rd edition), Paracetamol is the most frequent cause of liver failure.

Paracetamol is the most frequent cause of liver failure

Davidson's Principle and Practise of Medicine (23rd Edition)

Even in the European Journal of Pain, Paracetamol has been awarded as the most dangerous medicine in the world.

Most dangerous medicine in the world Paracetamol

European Journal of Pain
27 November 2014
https://doi.org/10.1002/ejp.621

So next time you experience fever, just follow the heat protocol as explained in the previous chapter and experience the magic of the self healing system of your body.

The self healing system of your body can be activated to reverse all kinds of lifestyle related diseases right from hypertension to heart disease and depression to diabetes through D.I.P. Diet explained next.

D.I.P. diet

The D.I.P. diet can be the fastest, safest and long lasting cure for more than 60 most commonly occurring diseases among humans. Even All India Institute of Ayurveda (under the ministry of Ayush) has conducted clinical trial (TRI/2018/016654, registered on 13/12/2018) for D.I.P. diet, under the guidance of Dr. S.K Gupta (HOD, Department of Shalya Tantra). The research scholar of the trial Dr Monika Sodhe reported a clear cut evidence of benefit in case of the back pain (the primary purpose of the study), the improvement is noted in terms of Thyroid, Blood Sugar, Blood Pressure etc as well.

In fact, in the last 15 years of my clinical practice in India, Vietnam (since 2014) and Malaysia (since 2017), millions of patients suffering from various illnesses have adopted the D.I.P. diet. The time line of reversal of disease based on these feedback of the patients and also my case study reports is presented in the tabular form on the next page. You will observe that as soon as a patient switches to a DIP diet, the disease reversal can be as fast as within 24 hrs to 72 hrs for diabetes and may range up to 8 months for disease like cancer, asthma, kidney diseases, skin diseases etc.

VIP Diet → D.I.P. Diet	
24hrs to 72hrs	Diabetes
3 days to 1 week	High Blood Pressure, High Cholesterol, Intestinal disorder
1 month	Obesity, Heart Diseases
2 month	Thyroid Disease
6 month	Cancer, Asthma, Arthritis
8 month	Skin Disorder, Kidney dysfunction, Liver disorder

STEPS TO DESIGN YOUR PERSONALIZED D.I.P. DIET:

Step-I

Till 12 noon, eat only fruits of 3 to 4 types including mango, banana, grapes, etc.

Minimum amount to be consumed = Your body weight in kg × 10 = ...gm

For example, a 70 kg person should consume atleast 700 gm of 4 types of fruits before 12 noon.

Step-II

Always eat your lunch/dinner in 2 plates. Plate 1 andd Plate 2

Plate 1 should consist of 4 types of vegetables like carrot, tomato, radish and cucumber etc. in raw form.

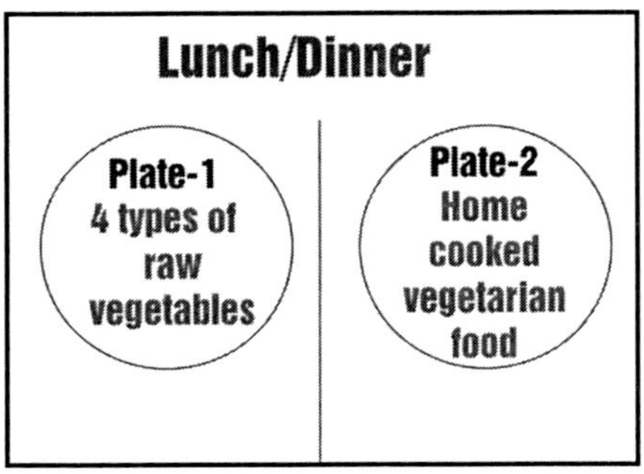

Minimum amount in Plate 1 = Your body weight in kg × 5 = ………... gm

For example, a 70 kg person should eat at least 350 gm of 4 types of raw vegetables.

Plate 2 should consist of home cooked vegetarian food with negligible salt and oil.

First finish eating from plate 1 in accordance with the above calculation, then take from plate 2 as much as you want. The rules for lunch and dinner are the same; however, you must remember to finish dinner by 7 pm.

Step-III

To Avoid	Snacking
1. Packed food	1. **Soaked nuts:** Your wt(kg) =......gm (For 70kgs person about 70gms of nuts in a day)
2. Refined food	2. **Fruits:** Plenty
3. Dairy food/Animal foods	3. **Coconut water:** As you like
4. Nutritional supplements	4. **Hunza Tea:** As you like
5. Avoid drinking tea/ coffee specially before lunch	5. **Sprouts:** Your Wt(kg)=.....gm
6. Never eat after 8pm	6. Coconut: As you like
7. NSAID's	7. Sunshine: 45min

You may need to modify and customize the above standard D.I.P. diet based on your symptoms/medical conditions and age.

Let every morning be the Hunza Morning

If you have decided to pick only one of my suggestions for the sake of your health, then take this suggestion:

Stop consuming tea specially, morning tea. The early morning tea makes the inner lining of your intestinal wall acidic, as after a long night of fasting your stomach is empty and craving for food. An acidic stomach on a regular basis is the single biggest cause of all kind of inflammatory and lifestyle diseases including arthritis, Diabetes etc.

How to stop craving of tea ⟶ Switch to Hunza Tea

Hunza Civilization: Hunza people are the Indians living at extreme northwest of India in Hindu Kush range. They are known to be one of the world's healthiest civilizations, often living up to the age of 110 years.

How to prepare Hunza Tea (serves four):

Ingredients:

- 12 Mint leaves(Pudina)
- 8 Basil Leaves(Tulsi)
- 4 Green cardamom (Elaichi)
- 2 gm Cinnamon (Dalchini)
- 20 gm Ginger (Adrak)
- 20 gm Jaggery (Gur)

Instructions:

- Take 4 cups of water in a tea pan
- Add all ingredients, simmer it for 10mins
- Add a dash of lemon juice and serve hot or cold

For those who are too lazy to collect the above ingredients (to make their own hunza tea) may order

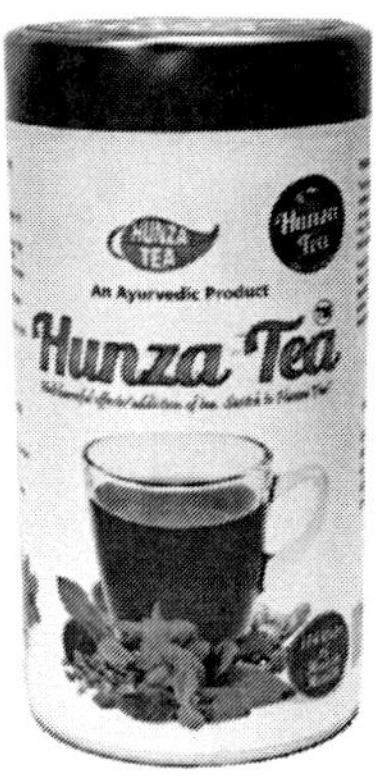

114 Cups of Hunza Health

₹ 400/-
(Including Courier charges)

You may place your order at:

Dynamic Memory Pvt. Ltd.
B-121, 2nd Floor, Green Fields,
Faridabad (Haryana)
Mobile No.:+91-9312286540,
E-mail: biswaroop@biswaroop.com

Log on to www.biswaroop.com/shop to buy products